LIVES AND DOLLARS

LIVES AND DOLLARS

The Story of Today's Research

By

JOHN D. RATCLIFF

Essay Index Reprint Series

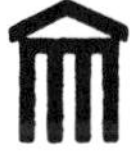

BOOKS FOR LIBRARIES PRESS
FREEPORT, NEW YORK

ACKNOWLEDGMENT

The author wishes to make grateful acknowledgment to the editors of *Collier's, Hygeia, McCall's, Reader's Digest, Survey Graphic, The American Mercury* and *This Week* for permission to reprint material which first appeared in those magazines.

PREFACE

"Science is the soul of the prosperity of nations, and the living source of all progress. Undoubtedly the tiring discussions of politicians seem to be our guide —empty appearances. What really leads us forward is a few scientific discoveries."

. . . LOUIS PASTEUR

To most people the world of the future looks dark indeed: a place of war, economic disruptions, and widespread poverty. To such notions the scientist says . . . "Absurd." Look ahead of the immediate haze, he says, and see a world quite unlike the one we know. It is a place where children aren't crippled by polio, and their parents aren't destroyed by cancer. It is a place where infants that survive the rigors of birth will live to be a hundred; a place of bountiful food, undreamed of leisure, unlimited atomic power.

As the architect of this Utopia, the scientist sees no necessity for war. After all, he asks, isn't war mass brigandage; an effort of one group to take desirable things from another group? If science can supply all needs, why fight?

Rank optimism, the reader may object. But think! Is it any more optimistic than the promise of today's life would have been to a man living in the 17th century; a man bitten by poverty, faced with periodic famines, and cursed with smallpox, typhus and plague? No. We will probably be nearer right in the end if we accept the scientist's picture of the future.

Louis Agassiz stated that every scientific truth goes through three stages: "First, people say it conflicts with the Bible. Next, they say that it has been discovered before. Lastly, they say that they have always believed it."

This is only partially true. As a rule people are badly informed about the happenings in research laboratories. So they don't discuss them at all. In 1903 they were more interested in Theodore Roosevelt's tailor-made revolution which resulted in the creation of the Republic of Panama, than they were in the activities of the Wright brothers, or the work of a lanky mechanic in Detroit who had the crazy notion that he could put a nation on wheels. A few years before this everyone followed the play-by-play account of a nearly forgotten Cuban revolution; but paid no heed to a 20-year-old Italian boy who that year began to send radio signals from his father's farm in Italy. Even in the enlightened year of 1935 we talked endlessly about the Supreme Court and about Ethiopia's fight—and passed over young Gerhardt Domagk's discovery of the sulfa drugs which were destined to save hundreds of thousands of lives.

Things of this same order are happening today: things which will still be shaping men's lives when the second World War has taken a small corner in the dusty pages of history; and New Deal reforms have assumed the importance of the Polk administration's tariff policy.

In this book we will see some of this scientific work in progress. To the reader the individual jobs may appear unrelated, and in a sense they are. They are merely isolated skirmishes in a broad frontal action. Yet they have a common aim: the saving of lives, or, in the case of industrial research, the saving of dollars.

CONTENTS

PART I

PART II

PART I

CHAPTER I

MADISON'S MIRACLES

Officially, the men who work in the ancient yellow brick building are horse and cow doctors. They are concerned with liver flukes, cow diseases, and things that give hogs the droops. Officially, that is. Actually, their work extends everywhere: into the home, hospital, delivery room.

This is the group of bio-chemists at the University of Wisconsin's College of Agriculture; a band of disease fighters whose work has touched every one of us in one way or another. They have found how to keep the bones of our children from bending with rickets, discovered the missing link in the picture of anemia, how to prevent that weary misery of the share-cropper which we call pellagra.

The staff is studded with great names: names recognizable wherever alert men are on the job of saving human life. There is Steenbock, tall, thin, slightly nasal voiced; Hart, gentle, fatherly, wise; Link of the towering intellect and the bizarre dress—tomcat bow ties, shorts, and sometimes bare feet. And there is Madden, Elvehjem . . .

The name Conrad Arnold Elvehjem has a glacial, academic sound. It sounds like a grim visage (a visage with whiskers), and like a pair of prepare-to-meet-your-Maker eyes. Actually, Connie Elvehjem is young—39. Being pure Norwegian, he is naturally blond. At a casual cocktail party meeting you would put him down as a prosperous young banker or business man. But never as the man who whipped one of the earth's ancient ailments.

Elvehjem—pronounce the letters L-V-M and you will have the pronunciation of his name—was born on a 120-acre dairy farm 10 miles out of Madison. More or less as a matter of course he went to the state university and also, as a matter of course, decided to study agriculture. Once there, he sensed the excitement of the chemistry laboratory and the great nutrition researches in progress. Cows, pigs and chickens couldn't compete with such heady stimuli. He forgot about plans to be a farmer.

After a long educational wind-up here and in England, the research project he staked out for himself, when he came home to a Wisconsin faculty job, sounds singularly unimpressive. He would study liver. But before making any decisions about how impressive or unimpressive this is, let's see a few facts. True, liver looks very sorry indeed as it lies in a drippy pool on a butcher's counter. Actually it contains as many problems as can be posed by the moons of Saturn or by the fragments of matter within the atom. It is a storehouse of vital food factors, all hidden so thoroughly that they require tortuous amounts of work for their finding.

Liver, it was known, would save lives of people suffering from pernicious anemia. And it would cure that slow death of the share-cropper: pellagra. Why it cured pellagra no one knew. No one had taken the trouble to isolate the chemical magic responsible. This was the job Elvehjem launched upon.

All vitamin work follows a pattern. First, a research animal —a guinea pig, rat, mouse, dog or chick—is selected. It is fed a diet of *pure* foods whose chemical composition is known: starch, sugar, casein (the milk substance from which cheese is made), salts, and known vitamins. Soon a deficiency manifests itself. The mouse stops growing, the chick gets ruffled feathers, or the rat has convulsions. Next step is to find some common food substance which will cure the condition: yeast, milk, liver. Then find what specific stuff it is in these foods that does the curative job. When you've accomplished this after several years' hard work you may—if you are lucky—have discovered a new vitamin.

This was the ambitious project the youthful Elvehjem staked for himself. Somewhere in liver there was a hidden substance which would cure pellagra. It was like looking for a needle in a stadium full of hay. Because of cheapness and ease of handling, he selected chicks as his research subjects. He fed them a special diet and watched while growth slowed and stopped. Their heads became pinched, their feathers ruffled, and their eyes bleary. They had a marked dermatitis. Was this chicken pellagra? Elvehjem thought so but other workers in the field didn't agree. He had better start again. Still convinced that he was right about the chicks, Elvehjem did start again—this time with dogs.

He fed them a pellagra-producing diet. Month after month Elvehjem and his helpers searched for the miracle secreted in liver which would cure this awful sickness. Eventually they found it—it turned out to be a common chemical—nicotinic acid. In 24 hours' time it would cure the horribly bloated tongue and lips. It would brush the cobwebs from human minds. Thousands of people scattered over the world have benefited by this magnificent piece of work.

Elvehjem, of course, is delighted that he has provided doctors with a superweapon to fight acute pellagra. But wouldn't it be better to *prevent* the disease, he asks? He admits that it is impossible, on short notice, to educate the South's poor away from pellagra-producing diets. But couldn't nicotinic acid be added to the cheap canned stews which are consumed in such quantities? This much is being done by dogfood packers to protect against dog pellagra—called blacktongue.

It was a nice idea but the Federal Bureau of Animal Industry rejected it. Nicotinic acid, it was decreed, was an "unnatural" food. The decision rankled Elvehjem. He snapped: "Mightn't we logically ask, why improve diet at all? If we do people will only live long enough to die of old age. To me it is very ironic that more objections are raised to adding vitamins to foods, than to destroying them by new processing methods."

Why are such problems of human nutrition investigated by an agricultural college? What has human pellagra in Georgia to do with problems of agricultural chemistry in Wisconsin? To the detached eye of the research man there isn't a vast difference between a cat, rat, dog and man. Each is heir to many of the diseases and nutritional upsets of the others. So work in one field keeps spilling over into another. As a matter of fact, the Wisconsin work began with cows.

If credit for the laboratory's preeminent position can be given one man, that man is Dr. Edwin Bret Hart. He was born at Sandusky, Ohio, on Christmas Day, 67 years ago. As a young man he worked at the Agricultural Experiment Station at Geneva, N.Y. He is now head of the bio-chemistry department at Wisconsin. Hart—"The Old Man"—has a fringe of white hair, a pink complexion. He suggests a trusting cherub. Actually, he is as tough and doubting as a Marine top sergeant, so far, that is, as research work is concerned.

When he arrived at Wisconsin the whole science of nutrition was neatly packaged and put away by workers in the field. Purely a question of calories—oh, how they loved that word —they decreed. Give a man or an animal sufficient calories and he would be perfectly healthy. So? Why then, wasn't coal the ideal food? Surely it was full of calories—Hart spoke the word with a contemptuous inflection. No, no, he said, there was more to it than that. He demonstrated.

He took several cows and fed them enough wheat to supply all the calories they could use. They sickened, fur became patchy, and growth stopped. They gave birth to dead calves. Then he fed a second group corn containing an equal number of calories. They thrived. See, gloated Hart, there is much that we do not know. A good case could be made for nominating cow No. 570 to the Hall of Fame. She lived longest, yielded most facts, and set off a splendid chain of research with world-wide implications.

Hart talked this cow thing over with two prize pupils, both farm boys. One was a tousle-haired youngster from Kansas—Elmer Verner McCollum. The other was Harry Steenbock, lanky, blue-eyed, who hailed from Charlestown, Wisconsin. Both were destined to make history; McCollum by discovering the first vitamin (A); Steenbock by finding the method for commercial manufacture of rickets-preventing Vitamin D. But this is getting ahead of our story.

Somehow, said Hart, they had to get this problem into the laboratory. Mac—McCollum—had a suggestion. They couldn't have mooing cows cluttering up the cubbyhole work rooms. They had to have smaller animals. Perhaps the rat would also get this cow sickness when fed a wheat diet. Certainly worth trying, all agreed. So Mac hauled out old packing boxes, sawed them apart and nailed them together into rat cages.

At the start there was a little grousing among outsiders about this rat work. Farmers who paid for support of the place weren't interested in preventing rat diseases. True, said Mac, but it is possible—probable—that a rat would yield facts translatable to larger animals, and perhaps even to man. Thus the work began. A few years later McCollum moved to Johns Hopkins where he continued his rat work. He ultimately found that they refused to grow on a diet of pure foods with known chemical formulae; but that a butter-fat supplement would correct this. From butter he finally isolated Vitamin A.

Meanwhile, at Wisconsin, Hart and Steenbock were busy with their own rat colonies. They hit upon a teasing fact. If young rats were taken from their mothers at weaning time and put on a diet of cow's milk they developed a dreadful killing anemia within a few weeks! Odd, this. Milk was supposed to be such a perfect food.

At the time doctors were saying that iron would cure anemia; then changing the subject when it was pointed out that many patients died even though they got iron enough to give them magnetic properties. Hart and Steenbock weren't at all surprised when iron failed to halt the march of blood-thinning anemia in their rats. But if iron wouldn't work, what would?

On milk-plus-iron rats died with doleful regularity. But if the diet was supplemented with lettuce they lived! Here was a striking fact, something solid to work on.

Let's, said Hart, burn this lettuce to an ash in an electric furnace. That will destroy any organic material—anything containing carbon—and leave only minerals. Then we can try the mineral ash that is left. If it cured this rat anemia the problem would be narrowed. The ash worked! Surely and quickly it cured the rat anemia. The job was nearly over. The ash had a bluish tinge—that suggested copper. Hart recalled something else that had previously escaped him. Soft-shelled crabs were far more blue-blooded than any Boston Brahmin. In the case of these crabs copper seemed to perform the oxygen-carrying function in the blood that iron did with human beings. This bit of reasoning clinched the problem. Copper was the anemia-curing substance. Doctors everywhere snatched at this information; began curing cases of anemia that had previously been difficult or impossible to treat successfully.

When this job was completed, the lanky Steenbock turned to another problem. He noted that rats raised on certain restricted diets and kept in the dark developed rickets. The sun cured the disease. Similar observations had been made in India. Children of high caste Hindus, carefully kept indoors, had this bent-bone sickness which was rare among poor children, allowed to play in the sun. Perhaps if foods were treated with ultra-violet light, a sunray component, these foods would cure the ailing rats. Steenbock tried, succeeded. Such light rays were needed for the synthesis of Vitamin D.

He patented the idea and assigned rights to the Wisconsin Alumni Research Foundation. To date revenue from these patents has amounted to a million and a quarter dollars, all of which has gone for research. The Foundation spends $160,-000 per year at Wisconsin; just recently completed a new lab wing for the old bio-chemistry building—a place of superlatively clean dog kennels, air-conditioned rat rooms, and beautifully equipped laboratories.

While these great things were going on the research men didn't forget their farmer constituents. For them they provided the butter-fat test by which milk is graded. Dr. Karl Link knew dairymen were troubled with poisonous properties of sweet clover hay. He isolated the poison, and developed a method of curing hay to eliminate it.

Hart recently made a discovery of tremendous importance. Farmers rely on linseed, cottonseed and soybean cake—refuse left after oil has been pressed—to supply necessary protein in cattle diet. He discovered that cows would produce as much milk and steers would put on as much beef on a hay diet supplemented with urea. This is the white, crystalline, nitrogenous stuff chemical plants extract from the air. Available in huge quantities, it is used in peacetime to make plastics and fertilizers; and in wartime as a base for explosives. Hart's finding comes down to this: he has found how to fatten cattle on a diet of hay and air! This discovery is particularly significant to such fat-starved countries as Holland, Denmark, Germany, England. It is also important to Wisconsin farmers who spend $20,000,000 per year on cake foods. Urea would cost them only a third this sum.

Oh, the farmers know they get more than their money's worth. Probably nowhere else in the world would one find such a group of research-minded agriculturists. Each year on Station Day they come to the university to see research in progress. Last year there were ten thousand on hand! Try and duplicate such a heartening scene elsewhere.

The laboratory has had a brilliant past and is preparing for an equally impressive future. Scores of projects are in the works. Researchers are attempting to corner an elusive growth factor that might explain why some youngsters are big and husky, while others are not. They are on the trail of a "grass juice factor" which accounts for summer sleekness of grazing animals.

How has this group been able to produce so much and to have so many lines stretching into the future? To Dr. Hart it is rather simple. "Get likely young men," he says, "and give them the bit. Make them get into the laboratory, feeding, weighing, and tending their own research animals. Then, when you have taught them all you know, send them away. It broadens them to work in other laboratories."

Men from Wisconsin have gone off to study in the universities at Zurich, Utrecht, Heidelberg, Cambridge, Berlin and elsewhere. Then they come back to the Old Man. "We have," he says, "been able to push the curtain back a little."

The Wisconsin work was chosen for the first chapter in this book because it illustrates how one spark can set off a firecracker chain of research. At the start no man can know into what territory his wit and imagination will carry him; he can only humbly follow each new lead as it appears.

CHAPTER II

THEY NEED NOT DIE

THE young interne watched helplessly while life seeped from the infant that lay before him. Internal hemorrhage, cause of 25 to 40 per cent of all fatalities among the newborn, had claimed another victim.

Could nothing be done to stop this murderous bleeding? Was there no way of preventing this seepage of blood into the skull; seepage that at times killed, and at other times crippled or paralyzed victims so that they might better have died? Would this splendid science of medicine have to remain forever powerless to prevent such tragedy? The interne put these questions to an older doctor.

Was there, he asked, an outside chance that a newly discovered vitamin might help? Vitamin K it was called; and it had performed brilliantly in stopping the ghastly hemorrhages that attended certain types of surgery. Might this stuff also work on these infants, forced to face the rude shock of death immediately on entering the world? It was certainly worth a trial, said the older doctor.

The men who talked thus were Dr. Dupont Guerry, and Dr. William W. Waddell, Jr., associate professor of pediatrics at the University of Virginia. The proposed trial took place and the new vitamin performed splendidly. It stopped bleeding from a wound in a newborn baby within a few minutes. When it was administered routinely to 400 infants, bleeding occurred only four times. In 219 other cases where it was withheld, there were 23 instances of hemorrhage! The opening words of a new chapter of medical achievement had been written.

The life-and-death drama of clinical success frequently overshadows the story of painstaking research that was a necessary forerunner. Such is the case here. Infants in Charlottesville, Virginia, could not have been spared without a laboratory accident in Denmark several years earlier.

Henrik Dam, research man at the University of Copenhagen, was investigating means by which dietary fat is utilized. He was using newly hatched chicks as experimental animals. One morning he noted that a number of them lay dead on the cage bottom. Flecks of red spotted their down. A finger run through the feathers exposed a horrid network of hemorrhagic blood vessels. The chicks had bled to death.

The *whys* that constantly assault any research man worth his salt began to plague Dr. Dam. *Why* had these chicks died? They had been given excellent food and the very best of care. They were well on a healthy road leading to a broiling rack when this spontaneous bleeding began. Was it just an accident of the type that puts grey hairs in the head of a research man? Or was there a hidden significance?

It was only five years later that he was free to continue the investigation. All over again he began to feed chicks on rice flour, yeast, salt, cod liver oil and fish meal from which fat had been extracted. Right on schedule this new generation of chicks began to die like their predecessors. After two weeks on the diet which presumably contained all necessary vitamins, they began to seep blood into the skin, from internal organs and through pinfeathers.

Examination showed their blood to be almost completely lacking in prothrombin—one of the four substances essential to blood clotting. When it is missing in a man a minor cut can become a major tragedy. Frankly, Dam didn't know what connection there was between the diet and the bleeding disease. But some vital substance simply wasn't there. He worried along with his chicks and tried other foods on them. Hog liver, he discovered, would cure the tendency to bleed. So would alfalfa meal. These things, in other words, contained elements missing in the other diet. Dam gave this mysterious something-or-other a name: *koagulation* factor, or Vitamin K.

While these significant things were happening in Copenhagen similar work was progressing in California. A group headed by Herman J. Almquist in the poultry husbandry department of the University of California's agricultural school, had found this same chick bleeding disease. And they had found that it could be cured by *putrid* fish meal. Nice fresh meal made from ground up sardines wouldn't do the trick. This indicated that by some miraculous process the bacteria of putrefaction were able to manufacture Dam's K vitamin.

So, with these assorted and not too sensational facts, we have the raw material for a really epochal piece of scientific research. If the reader isn't weary of hopping about the globe, we will backtrack to St. Louis. The scene is a nondescript classroom in the old medical school of St. Louis University. A pleasant young graduate student named Ralph McKee is reading a paper before the Journal Club. The dozen or so members of the club bone up on some subject in current chemical literature, then report to the group. This saves all of them time in having to wade through masses of material.

McKee tells about the work with the chicks. His paper doesn't exactly put people on the edges of their chairs. But there is polite interest from all except one man: Dr. Edward A. Doisy, head of the medical college's department of biochemistry. Doisy is taut as a fiddle string: pulling nervously on his omnipresent pipe and not missing a word.

When McKee finished reading his paper Doisy summoned him to his office. A sharp cross-examination followed. Doisy asked for all the literature on the subject. That night he took it home with him. He read and re-read the publications until he could recite them by heart. Then he called his group together: MacCorquodale, Sid Thayer, Steve Binkley, and the fiery Joe Yglesias. The group, all of whom had their doctorates except Spanish-born Joe, listened while the master spoke.

This K substance, said Doisy, might have splendid possibilities. It would stop bleeding in chicks. As to where else it might lead anyone could guess. Finding it was going to be a tough job but they were going to try.

There was no inspirational quality in Doisy's talk to his group. He is as matter of fact as a loaf of bread. Certain things were known, certain others unknown. They were going to isolate this mysterious K stuff in its absolutely pure form; tame it and see what could be done with it. Or at least they were going to try.

Thayer, said Doisy, was to start finding out how to raise chicks. Before they were through he would probably be a master poultry husbandman. Prophetic words, these. Thirty thousand chicks passed through Thayer's hands. McKee, said Doisy, would see what possibilities he could find in the putrid fish meal. Binkley could work with alfalfa. Mac, Joe and himself would handle the chemical end and generally oversee all the work. Thus the search began; a search that started in 1936 and is now nearing completion.

The first job was to find something which would dissolve the vitamin out of the alfalfa; and out of the fish meal which gave off a stench to shame a glue works. Trial and error chemistry finally produced the product: petroleum ether, a dry-cleaning fluid.

There was but one way to test these substances which issued from the labs of McKee, Binkley and Doisy. They were handed over to Sid Thayer for assay on chicks. By this time Thayer's lab looked like a prosperous hatchery. As many as 1,500 chicks were on hand at a time. As new substances were delivered for testing, he would pry open a chick's beak. A hypodermic syringe would shoot the material directly into the crop. A few hours later he'd open a wing vein, draw a little blood, and test it for prothrombin.

Week by week the group got closer to their elusive prey.

Substances produced got more and more potent; and smaller amounts would magically stop the blood seepage from chicks. Might it also work with men? Work with them to stop hemorrhages? Answers to this came almost simultaneously from three groups—one in Iowa City, a second at the Mayo Clinic and a third in Copenhagen. All had made clinical trials with extracts of Vitamin K. In certain types of surgery this stuff acted as dramatically as it did with chicks!

Vitamin K, it developed, was a fat-like substance. And fats are digested in the intestines with the aid of bile, secreted by the liver. Therefore, let anything happen to the bile-producing apparatus of the body and Vitamin K could not be digested and absorbed into the blood stream where it was needed. When this happened the body lacked the stimulus necessary to manufacture prothrombin.

Many things can slow or stop delivery of bile to the intestines. Infection of bile ducts, gallstones, degeneration of the liver, strategically placed tumors all achieve the same end result. At such times surgery, or even relatively minor wounds can cause fatal bleeding.

Once clinicians had this knowledge, corrective procedures were apparent. Before operating, feed a patient extracts of K along with bile salts to aid absorption of the vitamin. This would fortify blood with clotting factors. In some cases surgeons purposefully neglected this precautionary procedure. They wanted to see how quickly this miraculous new tool would work. It developed that in the space of a few hours K would, in most instances, stop seepage from surgical wounds; and in even less time would stop hemorrhages that were formerly fatal.

These results, recall, were obtained with impure extracts. No one had yet been able to corner the pure vitamin. But Doisy's group was hot on the trail. Work took on a feverish intensity. Sundays and holidays merged with other work days and everyone kept lab hours of 8 A. M. to 11 P. M. This went on for months.

But no one complained about the hours. They were about through—or at least they thought they were. Week by week extracts got purer. Finally the workers got a yellow oil that was only a few steps removed from the pure vitamin. There was a little gloating. Then something happened. One morning Sid Thayer was running a routine assay with a chick and the oil—which represented over two years of killing labor—refused to work! Something had gone wrong!

Brows of all workers wrinkled into accordion pleats. Dammit, it *had* to work. But it didn't. There was only one explanation. In its pure form this crazy vitamin was apparently sensitive to light. Rays from sun streaming in through windows and from light bulbs at night had destroyed it. There was only one thing to do, Doisy said. Get roofing paper, cover all lab windows. Then start all over again.

That summer the place became a smelly inferno. McKee's percolating fish meal gave off a maddening stench. From working long hours in the semi-darkness the eyes of most of the group became painfully inflamed.

This second time no hitches appeared. After a little over a year's work the pure vitamin—a lemon yellow oil—was isolated. The group went on to determine its chemical structure and to synthesize it—make it artificially. By a curious coincidence synthesis was announced simultaneously by L. F. Feiser of Harvard and Almquist of California.

At present one of the greatest indicated uses for these substances is in management of childbirth cases. For reasons as yet unknown probably half of all newborn infants have abnormally small amounts of prothrombin in their blood. Whatever supplies they have are derived from their mothers. Since their own intestinal tracts are sterile it is impossible at first for bacteria to make an independent supply of necessary Vitamin K. The slightest injury to these infants during birth, or in the first few days of life can have fatal consequences.

Work aimed at reducing the number of these casualties is progressing rapidly. In some cases mothers are routinely dosed with Vitamin K for the last month of pregnancy; in others newborn infants are given precautionary doses immediately they are born. One of Guerry's first cases in Virginia indicates effectiveness.

Blood was removed from the nostril of an infant girl three days after birth. This indicated trouble. A puncture was made in the heel to draw blood for routine analysis. It took this blood eleven minutes to clot! Seepage from this wound continued for twelve hours. A tiny amount of Vitamin K was administered by mouth. Within a few minutes blood seepage from the heel wound stopped. Within 90 minutes clotting time was cut in half and continued to fall until it stood at a normal three minutes.

One question naturally occurs. Will Vitamin K remedy hemophilia, the bleeding disease of the Spanish royal family? Doisy checked this early in his researches. As expected, the answer was no. Hemophilia traces to a deficiency of a blood-clotting factor other than prothrombin.

Victory here would have made headlines but actual importance would not have been comparable to the successes already noted. Hemophilia is a rare disease. Bleeding in the newborn, and hemorrhage in the types of surgery mentioned are not.

Thus the story of K is more than just the story of another vitamin. The stuff is widely prevalent in diet and its lack appears only under special circumstances. It will never be a material which we will keep on bathroom shelves to gulp casually—and often foolishly—as we take other vitamins. Its use will be restricted to delivery rooms and surgeries, and its job will be to give life to those who otherwise would have little chance of survival.

CHAPTER III

FOOD FOR THE HUNGRY

THE great pioneers in the nutrition field set the stage: Mc-Collum fussing with his rats; Steenbock wondering why bones didn't bend if they got enough sunlight; Eijkman, the Dutchman, working in Java with the Oriental disease, beri-beri; Windaus, the magnificent intellect of Göttingen; and dozens of others.

They showed us how to cure diseases with chemical magic. Men on the verge of death were snatched back and made well again in a matter of days; and in some instances hours. Yet none of these great men seriously proposed that the human race should be fed from pill bottles. Nothing could substitute for a well-balanced diet. Yet—how could you get people to eat such a diet? How could you convince the share-cropper that his meal, meat and molasses would, in the end, kill him? How could you get him to plant gardens; and how could you win industrial workers away from meals largely composed of starches and sugars? In other words, how could you change the habits of 130,000,000 people to make them conform to the findings of a handful of researchers?

Think of that for a while, and try to puzzle out an answer. The problem was enormous and the way it is being solved is one of the very finest things that has ever happened in America.

Each day now one and a half million children are getting free noonday meals. They are growing up with vitamin-rich foods not encountered at home; learning the lessons taught by men whose names they will never know. Out of America's bounteous market of surplus commodities they are eating their way toward health and sound citizenship.

We have shed tears and money for the hungry children of Belgium and China. They are dramatic, and we like drama. But at the same time we have tolerated the specter of starvation at home!

Possibly the reader doubts. Nearly all of us allow ourselves the luxury of thinking that everyone eats well in this country. But the person who yields to these thoughts hasn't seen—as I have—the lusterless hair, dull eyes, and sunken cheeks of children in the cotton country, in the coal-mining regions of West Virginia, or in the slums of New York City.

And he hasn't tried to explain away shocking figures: draft rejects averaging 25 per cent; and seven times as much tuberculosis and three and a half times as much pneumonia as there should be, in lower income brackets. Bad diet causes more misery and death than all microbes put together.

The free lunch program for children attacks the problem at its roots. Sponsored jointly by WPA and the Surplus Marketing Administration, it represents an organized, large-scale effort toward lasting national defense.

Surgeon General Thomas Parran is the most articulate exponent of this assault on hunger.

"We are wasting money," he says, "trying to teach children with half-starved bodies and minds. Improperly nourished children can't absorb teaching. They hold back classes, require extra time of teachers and repeat grades. This is expensive stupidity, but its immediate cost is nothing compared to its ultimate cost in unnecessary sickness.

"Something like 9,000,000 school children are not getting a diet adequate to promote health and well-being. My proposal is simply this: that we allow none of these children to starve.

"Science has given us a new definition of starvation. A child can eat its fill of a badly balanced diet and starve just as surely as a child with no food. There are ten cases of sub-clinical pellagra for each one that reaches a doctor. Only rarely do we encounter an outbreak of scurvy such as Maine had a short while ago, yet surveys indicate that a third of all children are dangerously low in scurvy-preventing Vitamin C. Latent malnutrition is our greatest producer of ill-health.

"Like nearly fresh fish, nearly adequate diet isn't good enough. We should see that all children are maintained at a level which produces abounding health and vitality. Such a plan would pay incalculable dividends."

The present program of free noonday meals for school children began in the days of the Civil Works Administration, the original work-finding, relief-giving federal agency. Earlier, in some localities and on a small scale, there had been feeding of undernourished school children by teachers. When the federal agency took up the work it was planned to feed only children of relief families, but a check-up showed malnutrition prevalent at other economic levels. A child has far more rigid dietary requirements than an adult. He will wilt on a regimen of minerals and vitamins sufficient to maintain his father. So the program was enlarged to include all children needing food.

WPA projects now operate in every state except Delaware, where school cafeterias are privately operated. There are about 18,000 participating schools. WPA furnishes cooks, waiters, dishwashers. The Surplus Marketing Administration supplies foods bought to sustain falling prices.

When fruits and vegetables glut summer markets SMA starts purchasing. It dried or canned thousands of baskets of California peaches, for example, when a bumper crop threatened a price collapse. In 1939 it supplied school children with an astonishing quantity and variety of food; nearly 100,000,-000 pounds, valued at $7,000,000. A few sample figures: 5,000,-000 pounds of butter; 1,000,000 dozen eggs; 17,000,000 pounds of citrus fruit and juice; 31,000,000 pounds of apples; 6,000,-000 pounds of peaches. A third to a half the foods on school lunch programs are supplied from these surpluses, the rest representing local contributions.

Each project must have the sponsorship of some tax-supported body—a state welfare department, a board of education. But help from a public-spirited local organization—Kiwanis, Rotary, Parent-Teachers—is often necessary to provide cooking equipment, dishes, or foods to supplement those supplied free by the SMA.

Parents in rural communities have been quick to sense the importance of a hot, well-balanced lunch for their children. If the one-room school had no facilities for preparing food, fathers have contributed time and lumber to build a kitchen and dining room, build tables, benches, repair old stoves.

Teachers are glad to assume responsibility. They have seen slow death in lunch pails: the corn-bread spread with lard; the flour-and-water biscuit containing a slice of sweet potato; the hoe-cake smeared with molasses. They have even seen children bring empty pails to school and go off alone at mealtime so that others wouldn't witness their poverty. At times on their own responsibility they have asked food contributions from more fortunate parents to supplement government donations. One parent supplied a beef on the hoof, which teacher and children butchered! In small rural schools, lunch cooked on the heating stove is served at the desks.

Some progressive rural schools have their own garden and canning projects, one Missouri county putting up 57,000 cans of fruits and vegetables. Schools have even raised their own pigs!

Cities generally use huge central kitchens, where food is prepared and delivered by truck to the schools. New York City has possibly the world's largest kitchen, servicing four of its five boroughs with 90,000 meals per day. Five hundred workers and 52 trucks are employed.

Where schools are equipped with cafeterias, and there are children needing hot lunches but not able to pay for them, WPA supplies extra help and SMA donates extra supplies.

There is one basic rule: no segregation of payers and non-payers. An empty stomach can't be a social stigma. Those unable to pay are given tokens resembling coins, or tickets.

Menus are prepared by trained dieticians. Samples: beef stew, macaroni and cheese, beets, whole wheat bread, orange, milk; scalloped salmon, green beans, whole wheat muffins, fruit gelatin, milk.

Ofttimes the foods offered are strange to the children. They are wary of them as you and I would be of the ten-year eggs delectable to the Chinese, or of the rancid yak butter found on the best tables in Tibet. One staple trick is to offer the new food only to children sure to eat anything given them. Others feel slighted and demand it. Another trick has converted thousands to grapefruit juice. At first it is heavily sugared, so that children will take it for its sweetness alone. Day by day the sugar content is lowered, and within a few weeks the juice is relished for its own taste.

This is a most important aspect of the free lunch program. It is giving the children a healthy appetite for protective foods —generally fruits and vegetables which they can grow in home gardens. It is winning a new generation away from meal, meat and molassses—the diet on which so many millions have slowly starved.

The children's response? Teachers report that the free lunch is the best truant officer yet found. Absences are generally cut in half and in one Illinois district they dropped 80 per cent! An Alabama principal notes that he can tell from attendance records which county schools serve free lunch. Afternoon fatigue is reduced, and the quality of class work is improved. There are fewer colds and less flu.

In a year's time half of 86,000 underweight children in Virginia were up to normal. In one 90-day period 63 underweight children in Georgia gained 210 pounds while a control group not eating the school lunches gained but 80 pounds. In a Southeastern Missouri county—a land of share-croppers, unemployed miners and timber workers—children gained an average of five pounds during the first month of the school program! In one Tennessee school all but two children were underweight when the free lunches were first served in the fall; by spring all but one were normal.

Still, this isn't a story of added pounds and increased stature. It's a story of brighter faces and brighter minds; a more secure present and a better future. It's the story of the Georgia child who had failed her work but then gained seven pounds and became an A student with the help of nourishing food. And of the Oregon girl who made a dramatic intellectual recovery after her teacher had decided she should go to a home for the feeble-minded. And of the fourth-grade Illinois boy who asked for a fourth bowl of soup. When an attendant jokingly suggested that he would burst, the child flushed. "This is all I'll have to eat until tomorrow noon," he said. For such children food is badly needed medicine.

A nation that properly protested the burning of surplus fruit and the slaughter of little pigs can find no objection to free lunches. Cost of the meals to the community is from 3 to 7 cents each, not allowing for the contributions of the Federal Government. Seven dollars would be a good average yearly cost per child. It costs $100 to give a child a year's schooling. One hot meal a day for badly nourished children is as good an investment in the future as any community can make.

Effects of the slow, insidious death we call malnutrition aren't dramatic. We can't from day to day see the slow bending of bones, the constantly falling resistance to disease, the gradual dimming of wits. We see only the end results—sickly, dispirited wrecks who might have been useful citizens. Then, often as not, we have the audacity to wonder about the worthlessness of some human beings!

Through motives purely generous and laudable we are concerned about our moral duty to feed a hungry Europe. The child in Nebraska can be quite as hungry as the child in

Wales or Brittany. We are today feeding a million and a half youngsters, but *there are five needing food for each one getting it!*

Surgeon General Parran would like to see free lunches provided *all* children, rich and poor alike, just as we provide free schools, books, transportation. He points out that even little Finland has seen the wisdom of such a policy. Agricultural surpluses would disappear, the health of the nation would rise to a new high. It is a challenging thought. "Through adequate nutrition," Dr. Parran believes, "we have it in our power to build a new race of people in America!"

CHAPTER IV

DEATH TO MICROBES!

THE vitamin researchers have taught us how to avoid the deficiency diseases by proper eating. Meanwhile, the medical research men have been making some remarkable advances. Discovery of the sulfa drugs will certainly rank with the greatest medical discoveries of all time. These innocent-looking white crystals have saved tens of thousands of lives. We shan't rehearse these stories here for by now they are too familiar to everyone. But an entirely new field is just opening up; one that looks quite as promising as the sulfa drug researches did five years ago.

This new work concerns the lowly grocery-store egg! These egg discoveries hold out promise of preventing some of the worst diseases in medicine's hall of ill fame. And isn't it even better to prevent a disease in the first place than to cure it after it has taken hold?

Lifesaving potentialities of the egg were discovered by Dr. Ernest W. Goodpasture, pathologist at Vanderbilt University's medical school. Goodpasture, 53, a veteran of research in cancer, flu, rabies, and other diseases, had undertaken a project with fowl pox—the chicken disease farmers know as "sorehead." It is caused by a virus—a microbe invisible even to microscopes.

Goodpasture was looking for a means of growing this virus; a means of getting it into the laboratory where he could watch it, work with it and see what tricks might be done with it. This step is always first in the study of any disease, and frequently it is one of the most difficult. The microbe of this sorehead sickness was no exception. It had to be fed and nourished to survive. Discovery of a tempting diet was the problem. Beef broth, agar and other microbe foods were passed by. The microbe went on a hunger strike and died.

By chance—happy chance that already has probably saved several thousands of lives—Goodpasture decided to try an egg diet. Pumping an old-fashioned dental drill with a foot treadle, he bored a hole in one end of a nice fresh egg. With a hypodermic syringe, he squirted virus through this minute opening. Then he put the egg in an incubator and waited. Nothing happened. The virus still acted like a balky child.

Undiscouraged, Goodpasture set off on another track. Perhaps a fertile egg would be tempting. Viruses, he knew, liked *live* tissue. The chick embryo might be just the meal. This turned out to be a brilliant hunch. The stuff did eat, grow and reproduce. A few chicks hatched bearing nodules of the disease! Then he chipped away bits of shell, inoculated the embryo and installed a minute window over the shell opening. Now he could actually see the virus at work; see it forming the nodules of this sorehead disease!

All this was academically interesting. But no one—save poultry raisers, and perhaps a few chickens—was going to shout with joy. Fowl pox wasn't that important. Still, implications of the work were tremendous.

To make a disease-preventing vaccine one must get quantities of the microbe responsible. Once obtained, they are killed or weakened so they can be shot without risk into a man. Inside the body they stimulate the blood into producing protection. Shots of this nature save us the grief of smallpox, typhoid fever, rabies and other diseases.

The essence of the problem, therefore, is to get bacteria by the billion, virus by the pint. This means providing food and warmth so they will grow the large families necessary. Some organisms—like the typhoid bacillus—get along quite well on beef broth. But the viruses—causers of thirty-odd ailments—demand live tissue. These microbes are responsible for such dreaded diseases as infantile paralysis, measles, sleeping sickness, and yellow fever.

Until a few years ago there was but one method of producing them—in the bodies of experimental animals. The virus of infantile paralysis would grow in monkeys. Yellow fever would grow in mice, and distemper in dogs. This was fine but far from satisfactory. In the first place the virus would likely kill the animal before any truly rich concentrations were reached. There was also the omnipresent chance that the virus would be contaminated by microbes of other diseases.

Goodpasture, a careful, cautious scientist, went on record. "We could," he said, "appreciate the great potential usefulness of a living host so easily obtained, so cheap and so uniform as the developing egg and at the same time so free of infectious agents." This was unbridled enthusiasm coming from a research man; a scholarly way of saying, "We've got something here."

Would these chick dinners tempt viruses of other diseases? Researchers in dozens of other laboratories wasted no time finding out. They went shopping for incubators, electric candling devices and other equipment.

Step out to Hamilton, Montana, to view some of this work that followed Goodpasture's pioneering. Hamilton is a small town in the Bitter Root Valley—scene of a chain of medical discovery that led to the conquest of Rocky Mountain spotted fever. This fulminating sickness, spread from wild rodents to man by ticks, killed as many as 75 per cent of the ranchers, surveyors and sheep men it struck. It also killed six researchers assigned by the United States Public Health Service to find its cause and cure. Eventually they did find a preventive vaccine.

But it had its drawbacks. It was expensive, difficult to make. The procedure was also highly dangerous. As already mentioned, the first step in making a vaccine is to get a rich culture of the microbe that causes the disease. In this case the tick—which spreads the fever from wild animals to men—was selected as the host.

At the Hamilton laboratory of the Health Service, workers put young ticks under wire cages on the backs of infected guinea pigs. When they had sucked enough blood to give them the disease the ticks were plucked off with tweezers. Ground up, they represented the base for a vaccine.

Possibly the microbe of this disease could be grown in fertile eggs—the way Goodpasture had done with the fowl pox. This thought occurred to Dr. Herald R. Cox—he is 33—researcher in the Hamilton laboratory.

Cox selected a few fertile eggs, punched holes in them and dropped in a small amount of the microbe of the lethal fever. Three days later the embryos were dead, killed by the microbes! This was food that appealed. Cultures were splendidly rich, as rich as the very best tick brew. This was a promising start.

Cox went on to extract these embryonic tissues and grind them up. Then he added salt water and whirled the mixture in a centrifuge to take out any solid matter. Next he added formaldehyde to kill the microbes. Would this vaccine work? Guinea pigs, faithful little creatures, would tell the story.

Over and over again Cox tested the new vaccine. Scores of guinea pigs went through the routine, surviving jolts of the microbe that should have killed them many times over.

When it was evident that this new stuff, cheaply and simply made, was successful, Cox turned to a similar disease, European typhus. Typhus—not to be confused with typhoid fever —is credited with having killed more human beings than any other disease. This 20 to 70 per cent fatal sickness is spread by body lice. During the first World War it killed over 3,000,000 Russians and held the Austrian army out of Serbia for months while the troops waited for the epidemic to run its course.

Here again a vaccine was available—in fact, two vaccines. But they, too, were difficult to make.

Using the technique that he had devised for Rocky Mountain spotted fever, Cox inoculated eggs with typhus. A rich culture resulted, and he went on to prepare vaccine from it. After satisfactory tests on laboratory animals, 2,500 doses for human beings were prepared. In special ice chests they went by plane to New York, boat to Italy, train to the sub-Carpathian region in Northern Hungary.

This area was chosen because Polish refugees were piling through mountain passes, bringing with them the disease, which had broken out in the German-occupied territory. Selected people among the population of three villages got vaccinations; others served as controls. Result of these trials will sooner or later tell the story. Glowing word it will be if the modest egg can whip the hulking killer, typhus. And lab work indicates that the story will go that way.

While this work was progressing the International Health Division of the Rockefeller Foundation was investigating the possibility that the egg might play a heroic rôle against yellow fever. Workers found that a fertile, six-day egg made perfect food for the yellow-fever virus. The virus ate heartily, and thrived, and within three days the egg contained enough microbes to launch a good-sized epidemic. From present indications vaccine made from such eggs is the most powerful weapon ever devised against the yellow death that stalks the hot belts of Africa and South America.

The most magnificent results to date with the egg vaccine have come not from a disease of men, but from a disease of horses. This is the horse sleeping sickness that bears a jaw-dislocating name: equine encephalomyelitis. Four years ago this disease swept through the horse herds of the country with unprecedented fury. It struck 170,000 animals. In some districts it killed as many as 90 per cent of those that got this paralyzing malady.

It reappeared in 1938 with even more disastrous results.

Furthermore, on this second visitation, the disease—probably mosquito spread—took a sideswipe at the human world. In an outbreak in Boston it killed 75 per cent of those stricken; left most of the survivors with such severe mental disorganization that they might better have died.

An old vaccine, made from brains of infected horses, was impotent against this killer. Egg work began at two places: Dr. Ralph W. G. Wyckoff of Lederle Laboratories carrying on one part of the project, Dr. J. W. Beard of Duke University the other. First tested on guinea pigs, the new vaccine was marvelously potent. It protected guinea pigs from shots of potent virus containing a thousand times the lethal dose!

Girls working in the Lederle Laboratories began inoculating 35,000 eggs a day and harvesting virus from the same number. Millions of doses of vaccine went out to make an astonishing record. Not one failure of the vaccine has been recorded!

These pieces of research which we have already examined are sufficient to cover the somewhat lowly egg with glory. But from present indications work has barely begun. Dr. Wendell Stanley of the Rockefeller Institute announced recently a new egg-grown vaccine which prevents measles. Viruses which grew haltingly or not at all in other media grow well in fertile eggs —thereby providing the base for lifesaving vaccines. It has been shown that at least 25 viruses will reproduce in eggs. Tragically enough, the one that causes infantile paralysis isn't among these.

Already research men are thinking of incubators in terms of saved lives, rather than in terms of broiled-chicken dinners. Thanks to them, people in Brazil are escaping the yellow death of the jungle, and people in Hungary aren't having to face the prospect of typhus. In the United States the incubator has removed the threat of a horse sleeping sickness which puts people in cemeteries or madhouses; and is holding out the alluring promise of protection against that ancient pest, the common cold. Altogether, these new egg tricks are fine indeed—much better than the one Columbus did.

In the following chapter we will see in detail how Good-pasture's discovery led directly to the most promising weapon against influenza yet discovered.

CHAPTER V

WHOLESALE DEATH

THE last epidemic of killing flu made grim history when it swept the earth in 1918. The next, now due, may leave a different record. For it will furnish a proving ground for a new vaccine; a vaccine that appears capable of whipping this 20th-century counterpart of the Middle Age plagues. It was discovered at the Rockefeller Foundation in New York. The vaccine came into being only after a superb accident had happened; one of those accidents that come along occasionally to give a researcher a hand-up over an apparently insurmountable problem. But let's get to the scene of action.

Dr. Frank L. Horsfall, Jr.—a medical man devoting his life to research—peered through the glass door of a ferret cage. The ferret stared back, murder in its eyes. This wasn't right. The wretched animal should have had a runny nose, aching muscles and fever. It should have been stretched on the cage floor, sick with flu.

Horsfall, 34, dark-haired, good-looking, pleasant, had infected the animal. Hands protected by heavy leather gloves, he had held up the flashing, writhing bundle of sharp claws and teeth, and carefully dropped influenza virus into its nostrils. By all rules it should have been miserably, wretchedly, beautifully sick within a few days. But it wasn't. Either there had been a bad slip-up or something momentous had happened.

Momentous was the answer. That healthy ferret with the evil eye was the tip-off on the new vaccine. It is quite possible that this shot-in-the-arm stuff may soon be saving us from something more dangerous than bombs. There is every chance that it holds the solution to history's greatest murder mystery.

Flu isn't an ordinary disease. It is elusive, subtle and complex; really a connoisseur's disease. For one thing, it isn't caused by a bacterium that can be easily housebroken to laboratory procedures. The flu bug won't eat the beef broth that nourishes microbes of typhoid fever and other diseases. And it can't be stained pretty colors and observed under the microscope.

Influenza is caused by a virus.

To see what kind of havoc this tough little customer can create, glance for a moment back to the pandemic of 1918–19. Possibly you've forgotten how terrorized people wore flimsy gauze masks; and how relief workers carried baskets of groceries to poor families only to find that coffins were needed. Or how people greased themselves, drank hot lemonades and prayed—to no avail. The black night rider slipped past all barriers.

A trader took the pestilential death to Point Barrow, north of the Arctic Circle. A rust-pocked freighter, a common laborer of the seas, put in at Upolu and Savaii, islands in the Samoan group. Within a few weeks a quarter of their populations were dead! Man's most studied efforts at killing, as expressed by four years of world war, looked feeble in comparison. This sudden death destroyed twenty million human beings!

After cutting its lethal swath across the earth the flu, which comes three times each century, disappeared. It left no clues —no positive medical knowledge—behind. It wasn't until much later that two brilliant groups of research men, one in England, one in the United States, began to inch their way through the darkness.

One worker has suggested that medical research is very much like children piling boxes against a wall. It is possible to see over the top only when many pieces of good, solid work have been piled one on top of the other. So before we get back to Horsfall and his stubborn ferret, let's examine some of the highly interesting boxes at the bottom of the pile.

Were we to try to put our finger on the date marking the beginning of the big push on flu, that date would be 1933. That year a group of British workers headed by Frederick Playfair Laidlaw (he became Sir Frederick before his tragic death two years ago) made nuisances of themselves in London hospitals.

Laidlaw and his co-workers—Christopher Andrews, Wilson Smith and H. C. Stuart-Harris—propped flu patients up in their beds. Then they'd hose their throats out with a syringe and collect the drippings in a pan. Surely, they reasoned, if the flu microbe was anywhere it would be in these throat washings.

Back in the Mill Hill Laboratory, maintained a few miles out of London by Britain's National Institute for Medical Research, they shot this throat juice into all sorts of experimental animals: rats, mice, guinea pigs and even that fabled creature of song—the hedgehog. The animals stubbornly refused to get sick. Then Laidlaw had another hunch. In his earlier work on canine distemper—which led to the vaccine used today to protect our dogs—he had employed the ferret. Possibly this miserable creature, hateful to all research men because of its filth, bad temper and extreme susceptibility to disease, could be infected with flu. The group, said Laidlaw, would try the nasal passages because flu seemed to enter the human body by this route.

They knew that if this thing worked they would have taken an enormous stride forward. They would have cornered this violent death in a single animal where they could watch it, fret over it, and perhaps get some real facts about it.

Laidlaw filtered the throat washings the group had collected in hospitals. The filter would strain out any bacteria—and the stuff that went through would be—what? Laidlaw didn't know. He hoped it would be virus—the virus of influenza. With a blunt syringe he installed a few drops of this elixir of death in the nose of a squirming ferret. Then the group sat back to wait. It wasn't a long wait—only 48 hours. Then one ferret got sick with a disease that looked like flu! Younger members of the group enthused. They had flu cornered in a research animal! It would be very easy from this point on. Laidlaw, patient and careful, curbed their enthusiasm. What made them think this was flu? Certainly it looked like that unruly disease. But unfortunately, he said coldly, good medical research wasn't based on casual appearances and youthful enthusiasms. They had to *know*.

They passed this sickness—whatever it was—from ferret to ferret; and from ferret to mouse. Then, after a few months of this, a splendid thing happened. Stuart-Harris was examining a ferret one day when it let go a beautiful full-blown sneeze, right in his face! Two days later he was flat on his back with fever, headache, sore muscles—but he had an ear-to-ear grin on his face. The cycle was completed. They had passed flu from sick man to ferret, and back to man again. It was a virus disease. Now things were moving.

Flu researchers the world over had a hot scent and were now on the trail. Down in Australia, F. M. Burnet took a tip from Goodpasture. He found that flu virus would grow and thrive in fertile eggs.

This discovery gave researchers the ready source of infective material that they needed. It saved them the tedium of grinding up lungs of mice killed by flu; or the nasal passages of ferrets.

Work of this sort, clever as sin, began to pop everywhere. A group of Russian workers in Moscow wanted to know what would happen if you dropped virus into human noses. They got a group of "volunteers"—whether or not they were captured from a passing street car the literature does not record. In any case the volunteers got the virus and got the disease.

Up at Harvard other men wanted to check on the belief

that flu is spread by sneezing. So they built a sneezing machine—a small glass-enclosed cage with an atomizing nozzle stuck in one side. Ferrets in the cage got flu after a couple of blasts of the atomizer. Further work with high-speed cameras and other equipment indicated that droplets are expelled from the mouth of a sneezer at the rate of 100 miles per hour; and that flu microbes in the droplets float in the air, well and happy, for as long as half an hour!

Meanwhile, the Rockefeller Institute in New York had its own problems. Dr. Thomas Francis, Jr., pink-faced, cherubic, confirmed the work of Laidlaw and began hunting virus strains of his own—in Alaska, Puerto Rico, Philadelphia. He noted that all strains were not alike; some were blustery and killing, others were meek and mild. As often as not an animal that was immune to one of these strains (by virtue of a recent attack of the disease) would not be immune to a second. Was flu, then, a disease like pneumonia, of which there are 32 types? It looked as if something of this sort might be the case.

Tommy Francis, friendly, gracious, a superb worker, chased flu microbes through the San Joaquin Valley in California and in labyrinthine depths of Brooklyn. He found that he could shoot the microbes of a certain strain—say Philadelphia 37—into the blood stream of an animal. Instead of getting the disease—as it would if the virus were dropped into the nostrils—the ferret reacted in quite the opposite direction. Somehow this potent juice caused the animal's blood to build antibodies—immune factors which fight off infection. After being vaccinated in this manner ferrets got high-grade protection!

Would a man react the same way when given shots of virus? Francis got a hundred volunteers and shot the flu juice into them. None of them had adverse reactions. Antibody content of the blood of nearly all of them shot up! It appeared that live virus vaccine would protect. Still, it had its drawbacks. For one thing, it was good only for a single strain. PR-8 recovered in Puerto Rico wouldn't protect against WS (named for Wilson Smith) found in London.

This was a discouraging fact with obvious implications. There were dozens of strains loose in the world and you couldn't vaccinate all of them. If you did, like as not an unknown one would drift in from somewhere to knock the vaccinated man over.

So things were left still pretty well up in the air. All researchers could do was wait for an epidemic. Then they could rush out, isolate the virus responsible, grow it in eggs and make a vaccine. No, this wasn't the answer. But this was the way things stood.

In the course of the seven previous years a tremendous assault had been made on flu. Shelves sagged under the literature that accumulated; but the key to the situation was missing. No man could be sure but what he would be among the twenty million that went to the graveyard next time flu took a world tour. Then a magnificent, history-making laboratory accident happened.

Dr. Frank Horsfall, who took over the Rockefeller flu work when Tommy Francis accepted a faculty job at New York University, noted that his ferrets were dying for no accountable reason. But a little investigation disclosed the cause: there was a lab epidemic of distemper, terror of all researchers who work with ferrets. This disease kills the animals surely and swiftly. It is costly—ferrets come at $4 each—and often erases months of tedious work already done on the animals.

Horsfall rushed to save what animals he could. His soft voice grew sharp as he prodded his four assistants to hurry: grind up lung tissue of animals that had died, whirl it in a centrifuge to remove solid particles and shoot this back into the hundred ferrets still alive. This would prod their blood into making protection. In a few days the epidemic eased; and in a week or so the decimated colony was safe. Horsfall heaved a mighty sigh of relief; then went on with the flu work.

Grasping better-tempered ferrets by neck and tail, and evil ones with forceps, he again started dropping virus in noses to infect the animals with flu. Then he sat back to wait for them to get sick, with the same assurance that a man looks to the West for the sunset. But they stayed contrarily, obstinately well! Horsfall bridled. Those creatures out of hell *had* to get sick. He was wrong as could be. They didn't have to at all. And they didn't. For some unaccountable reason the Stuka microbe that had always caused flu before wasn't working!

Worried, Horsfall checked his virus and found it still potent enough to kill mice. There was but one explanation. Somehow—he hadn't the slightest idea why—the combination of the flu virus from human beings and the distemper virus from dogs seemed to give ferrets wide-scale protection. It seemed—and here was a striking fact—to protect them from all types of virus on hand in the lab. Here was the overlapping effect that research men had sought for so long!

This thing had splendid potentialities. The Australian, Burnet, had shown how to grow virus in fertile eggs. This eliminated troublesome animals from the picture. One could shoot both the flu and the distemper virus into an egg, slip the egg into a nice warm incubator whose temperature was kept at 100°F. The microbes would grow and reproduce into a rich culture that could be used as the basis for a vaccine. There was but one catch to these pleasant, lulling thoughts. Would this combination virus vaccine protect men as it protected ferrets?

Horsfall inoculated various lab workers, checked their blood after a few days and found that average antibody content had shot up several hundred per cent! Such an observation is by no means conclusive proof that these men would ride unscathed through a flu epidemic. But it is the next thing to proof. One large-scale check indicated that people with many antibodies in their blood were only an eighth as likely to get flu as people with only a few.

What Horsfall needed at this point was a good, lusty flu epidemic.

While the mild, soft-spoken Horsfall didn't exactly wish anyone bad luck, it still wouldn't be altogether accurate to say that he was distressed by word which arrived from Puerto Rico. Flu had broken out. Working day and night, he and his helpers prepared thousands of doses of vaccine.

The finished stuff was rushed to Puerto Rico. Tragically enough, it got there too late. The epidemic, instead of growing and spreading, had petered out. No conclusions could be drawn from the few people who did get the painless shots in the arm. Then good news came from the West Coast—that is to say good news for the medical researchers. Flu was knocking people over by the tens of thousands, in California, Oregon, Washington, Idaho, Arizona and New Mexico. In some communities it was putting 20 per cent of the inhabitants to bed! It wasn't the killing flu like that of 1918 but, just the same, it was flu.

Horsfall hurried his vaccine to several California towns and vaccinations began. Results of this work won't be known until the statisticians make their tabulations—and they are remarkable for their leisure.

Epidemiologists are betting even money that London will have a severe outbreak. With thousands of people piled pell-mell into insanitary, badly ventilated bomb shelters and subways looking like termite tunnels, conditions are ideal for growth and spread of two diseases, meningitis and flu.

If the vaccine gets its big chance and proves to be successful, the final chapter will have been written in mankind's most costly, most lethal plague. Tomorrow's newspapers will be telling you how the tide is running.

CHAPTER VI

BULLY-BOY MICROBE

Tens of thousands of CCC boys have lined up before Army doctors who have charge of camp health work. Needle plungers send minute doses of a clear, colorless fluid into their arms. The boys know that these shots, which they volunteered to take, have something to do with pneumonia. The shots might protect them from the sullen fury of this killer disease. The doctor said that. But he stressed the word *might*.

Had he been in a talkative mood, the doctor could have added a great deal more to the story. He might, for instance, have mentioned that the organism that causes pneumonia is the killer supreme; that in the past it killed upward of 100,000 Americans every year. He could have suggested that a vaccine to keep people from dying of pneumonia would rank as the greatest achievement since Edward Jenner found how to save people from death or disfigurement at the hands of smallpox. Beside such an accomplishment, the doings of a Hitler or a Churchill would rank as very small beer indeed. To wind up his little sermon, the doctor would glance at the fluid in his poised hypodermic syringe. This stuff, he would say, looked like the most promising step yet taken in that direction.

In all probability the doctor said none of these things. Most likely his conversation was limited to two words: "Next man." So we will get along with the story here. Like all tales of medical research it begins a long way back. The spring of 1913 is our date.

Dr. William Henry Welch, who studied in Germany and came home to set up the first United States course in pathology at Johns Hopkins, was lecturing to a group of students. It was his famous Monday 12 to 1 course in bacteriology. Welch was going alphabetically through the students. He got to the F's. Turning to a chunky, tow-headed youngster, he asked: "What is virulence?"

The youngster fumbled miserably for a few minutes and then admitted that he didn't know. Welch smiled. "Neither do I," he said. He went on to explain. Nobody knew why one strain of microbe would be sure death and another of the same family would cause only relatively mild manifestations. If a means could be found of lessening virulence of any microbe strain, he added, that would be tantamount to controlling disease.

The young medical student who listened with fascination to all this was Lloyd Derr Felton, son of the Lutheran minister at Pine Grove Mills, Pennsylvania.

Felton was taking bacteriology and had decided to go into research. No better place to begin, he decided, than with the virulence of that particularly lethal microbe *Diplococcus pneumoniae*. If you could tame this one you would save lives by the million. Since then Felton has worked at the Rockefeller Institute, Harvard, Johns Hopkins, and, finally, at the National Institute of Health, the research organization maintained by the United States Public Health Service. For twenty-odd years he has worked almost continuously with the microbe which is shaped like a pair of linked berries.

There are 32 specific pneumonia bacteria. The casual eye cannot distinguish one from another, but delicate tests are available which will do the sorting job. Curative serums— made from blood of horses or rabbits which have been injected with heat-killed microbes—are available for most types. These serums are capable of cutting death rates in half. The magic new drug, sulfapyridine, is even more effective. It cuts the normal death rate of 25 per cent down to 6 or 8 per cent.

Superb as these weapons are, they are valuable only when

pneumonia has developed. The old question arose. Wouldn't it be better to prevent the disease in the first place? Most researchers thought so and have devoted an enormous amount of attention toward finding a vaccine that would be as effective as the protection we now have against diphtheria, tetanus, typhoid and smallpox.

Most of these efforts have been directed toward finding an antigen. Get that word fixed in your mind, for you are going to hear a lot of it from now on. Antigen is any substance that stimulates production of antibodies. It may be something in the structure of the bacterium or it may be a product of bacterial metabolism.

This material has rather miraculous qualities. It gives the body the kick that it needs to make it fight off bacterial invaders. It does this by stimulating human blood to produce antibodies. Antibodies in their turn usually kill off bacteria. This completes the suicidal daisy chain; the microbe carrying the seeds of its own destruction. Like traders passing out guns and liquor to Indians, so the Indians will come back and shoot them.

Very well, said research men everywhere, why not extract this antigen from bacteria and shoot it into men? Soon their blood would be swarming with protective antibodies. Whenever a microbic Goliath wandered in, these potent little Davids would swarm over him and there would be one less health hazard in the world. Antigens might represent the surefire protection all human beings wanted against disease.

On paper it was an enticing idea. But how could you operate on a microbe so small that it took twenty-five million of them, standing shoulder to shoulder, to cover an inch? It seemed preposterous but chemistry offered a way out. The chemical approach was to dissolve billions of bacteria and then work on the resulting batch of débris.

Using such a procedure, Drs. Michael Heidelberger and O. T. Avery, workers at the Rockefeller Institute, chipped off a fraction of the pneumonia microbe in 1923. The fraction, they found, was a complex sugar molecule—a polysaccharide. It wasn't, said the dark, scholarly Heidelberger, the antigen for which they had been searching. So this SSS (soluble specific substance) was more or less filed away. Then, in 1927, two German workers named Schiemann and Casper announced that SSS *did* look like antigen.

Felton, who had been working at Harvard along similar lines, flew off on this track. Microbes were stewed up into a witch's broth and SSS was extracted. The white, powdery stuff, which looked like ordinary table sugar, was dissolved in salty water and shot into the tail veins of mice.

The big moment came when Felton began inoculating mice with pneumonia microbes. If the antigen had worked—if it had caused the mice to build antibodies—they would survive. If it hadn't they would die. For such work the mouse is a superb subject. He has no immunity whatsoever to the bully-boy microbe which causes pneumonia. Incredible though it sounds, dilutions of culture containing but a single pneumococcus will kill a mouse!

Eighteen hours after being injected with the microbes the control mice began to die. These were the ones that got only the microbes—and none of the antigen. Felton waited impatiently. Thirty-six hours passed. This was the critical time. All mice in the control cage were dead. But those that had gotten antigen lived—lived despite the fact that they had gotten walloping jolts of microbes that should have killed them several thousand times over. The stuff that looked like table sugar did protect—protect mice, that is.

Lab assistants burbled with excitement. Not Felton. He is not the excitable type. All that had been done so far, he pointed out, was to save the lives of a few insignificant mice. And there were too many mice in the world anyway. There were a few mild protests. "Dammit, enthusiasm doesn't make facts," he snapped.

How much did this antigen increase the antibody content of mouse blood? How long did the protection hold up? How big a jolt of pneumococci would it fight off? Did it have any toxic qualities? Questions like these had to be answered with mice as the subjects before man could step into the picture.

For a while the laboratory fairly crawled with mice. There were mice with yellow dye on right forelegs, and mice with yellow dye on their backsides. Various markings told workers at a glance what combinations of antigen and microbes had been shot into the creatures. Work progressed at a feverish pace. Felton took time out at noon for a bottle of Coca-Cola and a handful of crackers—his usual lunch—but spent the rest of his time at a workbench. The day finally arrived when it looked safe to try antigen on human subjects.

Lab workers rolled up their sleeves. First they donated a little blood that would be tested for antibody content. Then they got shots of antigen. Another blood withdrawal two weeks later would show whether there was a large enough increase of antibodies to stave off pneumonia.

After their vaccinations, arms swelled painfully. Felton's puffed up like a sausage balloon and turned black and blue. (It developed later that these initial shots were four times too large.)

Two weeks later came tests that told the story. If the antigen had worked there would be a tremendous increase in antibodies in the blood and these antibodies would protect men against pneumonia. They would also protect mice. The test was simple enough. Blood was withdrawn from vaccinated lab assistants and whirled in a centrifuge to remove red cells. The serum, or "white" blood would contain whatever antibodies were present. If rich in this protection it would save lives of mice which had also been shot with killing pneumococci. Mice lived after receiving thousands of lethal shots of microbes. The antigen did give human beings protection.

The thing held out magnificent promise—promise that

people need no longer die at the hands of a cruel killer. But Felton was not interested in promises. He wanted facts and there was only one way to get them. It was readily apparent that thousands—perhaps hundreds of thousands—of people would have to be vaccinated. Only in this way would it be possible to tell the effect of the vaccine on the relatively small number of people that normally get pneumonia.

Before undertaking such a huge project, another thought occurred to Felton. Why not pick a few people predisposed to pneumonia, people who had had the disease several times, and try it on them? See if it would ward off future attacks? Thirteen subjects were selected for this experimental trial balloon. One youngster in the group had been sick with pneumonia thirteen times—every year since his second birthday. Inoculations for this series of patients began in 1929. No more pneumonia has appeared in the group since that date!

For his large-scale project Felton was presented with a nice problem. How could he get the thousands of subjects needed? And how could he follow them afterward to find what results the vaccine turned in? Why not use CCC boys? Since they lived under controlled conditions and had constant medical supervision they made ideal subjects. The all-important matter of records could be solved easily. Felton approached Army doctors. They were enthusiastic for a number of reasons.

In peacetime, pneumonia presents no particular problem to the Army. As a cause of death it ranks behind automobiles and suicide. But in wartime, pneumonia is quite another matter. With thousands of men crowded into hastily constructed barracks, pneumonia becomes a problem nearly as large as enemy bullets. In the World War, for example, the disease killed 19,000 American soldiers.

The Army promised fullest cooperation, and inoculations began in December, 1933. That year 3,000 CCC boys volunteered for vaccination. Case records were kept on a second unvaccinated group of 9,000 men. These were the controls.

Cases began to appear in the unvaccinated group—eight in all. Two of the boys died. Not a case appeared in the group that got Felton's vaccine.

Army men were enthusiastic, but Felton ripped into the figures. There were only 3,000 vaccinated men. Normally one out of 500 would have got the disease. That meant only six cases. The fact that six men, lost somewhere in that group, didn't get pneumonia meant precisely nothing. More likely than not, individual good health or good luck had protected them. It was a strange reaction from Felton. It was the scientist in him speaking. Wait until next winter, he said, and let's try again—with more men.

Vaccinations started with a new group the following November. This time there were 14,000 who got the shots, and 14,000 who didn't. In the unvaccinated group there were 23 cases of pneumonia and two deaths. In the vaccinated group there were no deaths. Thirteen men got the disease and five of these cases were extremely mild—not much more than a bad cold.

These figures pleased Felton far more than those produced in the previous year. Not for a moment had he thought—or hoped—that his vaccine would give complete protection. There was too much variation in individual reactions. But if it would radically reduce the case rate, and perhaps weaken the disease when it did strike, that would mark a highly gratifying start. The vaccine had done these jobs.

Vaccine for these cases had been made in Felton's own laboratory but facilities were not available for its production on a really large scale. So Army doctors asked him if he wouldn't set up operations in conjunction with their vaccine plant at the Army Medical School in Washington. This laboratory produces all the typhoid vaccine required by the Army. It is probably the cleanest spot on earth—as nearly bacteria-free as human ingenuity can make it.

The Army went to work in this fabulously clean place.

Buying prime beef in 200-pound lots, they stewed it into broth-food for pneumonia microbes. They harvested them by the billion and used chemical magic to chip off the wanted antigen. Doses of this stuff, packed in rubber-stoppered ampoules, went out to CCC camps all over the United States. The largest controlled experiment in medical history began.

Year by year the number of boys vaccinated rose. In the winter of 1937–'38 it was 111,000. In 1938–'39 it was 115,000 and in 1939–'40 it was 120,000. From these huge groups enough figures have developed to tell the story of the vaccine as it stands today. Among those inoculated, pneumonia occurs only half as frequently as it does with the controls; and the mortality rate among those who do contract the disease is lower. When it does strike, it is often mild.

From present indications the vaccine appears to protect for one to two years. So far as Felton is concerned, it is still far from satisfactory. "I want a 100 per cent efficient prophylaxis against pneumonia," he says. "One that works only half the time isn't good enough." So he is striving for perfection. He has cut out for himself a job of staggering proportions. To be perfectly straight about what he is up to at the moment let's understand one thing: there is a different antigen for each of the 32 pneumonia microbes. The vaccine so far has contained only antigen for types I and II. These account for over 40 per cent of all cases.

Although this vaccine has been specifically designed to prevent these two types, a curious overlapping effect has been noted. In some instances the vaccine appears to ward off types of pneumonia for which it is not intended, and in others it lowers the violence of the disease when it does occur. To Felton this overlapping effect indicates one thing. Perhaps there is a common denominator for all the antigens. Hidden somewhere in the complex sugar molecules there may be a simple chemical substance which will prevent *all* pneumonia.

The thought is enticing. Felton has begun the search.

Where it will lead no one can guess. Felton will not speculate but it appears possible that this common denominator will be the 100 per cent efficient prophylaxis he is seeking. If this search is fruitless there is yet another approach to a more efficient vaccine. Antigens for all 32 types can be mixed in one shotgun dose of vaccine.

As a corollary to this project, he is off on another job which is aimed at eliminating one of the objections to the vaccine as it stands today. Admitting its good qualities as proved by the CCC tests, how many people would be willing to take it? Assume that in a group of 500 people only one case of pneumonia will normally occur. Should all 500 undergo vaccination when it promises only half a chance for one of them to escape the disease? Felton says no. He is now attempting to perfect a skin test which will indicate *susceptibility* to pneumonia; just as the Schick test indicates a disposition toward diphtheria. By thus separating sheep from goats, the number of people requiring annual vaccination might be reduced materially.

These things—perfection of the test, and finding the common denominator of all the antigens—remain for the future. For the present the vaccine, which is not yet available to the general public, is turning in promising results. It has stopped epidemics in their tracks. One such case occurred in a boarding school in Virginia. The infirmary was filling rapidly and school authorities were sick with worry. The entire student body as well as the faculty got gentle jabs of vaccine and no more cases occurred.

Another time an outbreak occurred in a Massachusetts hospital for the insane. Eighty-four people went to the hospital with pneumonia and the outbreak appeared to be just getting under way. Then nineteen hundred people were vaccinated. After that only four new cases occurred. Three of these were people who had refused vaccination.

Chapters one and two in the long and disheartening story

of pneumonia covered the development of serum and sulfa-pyridine. These things save lives of people with the disease. Chapter three is the story of a vaccine. Admitting that Felton has a long way to go, he has at least made a start into this virgin territory.

CHAPTER VII

BAD BUG

THE story of Rocky Mountain spotted fever isn't an ordinary tale of medical research. It's one of the fabulous sagas of the trade. It's the story of the seven who died while looking for a means of prevention; and of the others who lived to carry the fight to final victory. And it's the story of a new serum which looks brilliant on paper, but must prove itself by saving the lives of human beings who contract the disease.

Before we take a closer look at the new serum let's rehearse a few facts about this ogreish disease. Not that we wish to frighten the reader. The chances of you or I getting spotted fever are thankfully remote. Most likely neither we nor our friends shall have occasion to call for this serum which appears to save. Yet it is consoling that it is on hand; consoling as a distant Pacific naval base which we shall never see, and perhaps never need. But there is always the chance . . .

The freight agent at York, Pennsylvania, would have been most grateful for it after he handled the shipment of raw furs. And so would the lady on Cape Cod who had plucked ticks from her dog. And the socially prominent Philadelphia banker who paid a horrible price for an afternoon's amusement de-ticking his prize cattle.

Spotted fever is spread by tick bites. Where ticks get this disease, which leaves them untouched, is not known. But it is known that they pass the fever microbe from mother to egg to baby ticks for dozens of generations on end. And it is known that on the average one out of every 500 ticks in nature carries this disease!

In the West the wood tick is the creature responsible for

spreading the disease to man; in the East it is the dog tick. The season for the disease starts in mid-March—when ticks are hungry from a winter's hibernation.

For trappers, surveyors and foresters spotted fever is, in a sense, an occupational disease. For others—hunters, campers, fishermen—it is a disease of recreation. On rare occasions it will strike at people who have as little to do with the woods as a café socialite. Why? How? These questions are generally impossible to answer; but somewhere in the picture there must be that minute, eight-legged killer. Mortality rates vary. In some areas (Idaho's Snake River Valley, for example) it kills only 5 per cent of those it strikes. In others it kills nine out of every ten that get it! This is true in the Bitter Root Valley in Western Montana, home port of spotted fever.

Chapter No. 1 in the conquest of this disease was written in the Bitter Root. In 1922, Dr. R. R. Spencer, a drawly-voiced, easy-going Virginian was assigned to the research job by the U.S. Public Health Service. Spencer knew of this violence with which he had been assigned to work; as dangerous as any known laboratory material. He knew that it had killed a promising worker at the University of Berlin; a researcher in Montana; a man of his own service; and an assistant of Hideyo Noguchi, that mighty mite of the Rockefeller Institute. (This was before it became Noguchi's turn to die of yellow fever on Africa's torrid Gold Coast.)

One fact stood out as a warning to the faint-hearted: *no lab man infected with the Bitter Root strain had ever recovered from spotted fever.* This was the situation when Spencer went to the Bitter Root to join forces with Dr. R. R. Parker. Parker worked for the state of Montana. Together they set up headquarters in a deserted brick schoolhouse at Hamilton; a tumbledown place decorated with an altogether too pretentious portico, and surrounded by a weedy, run-down yard.

As if to banish any lingering doubts as to the potency of this death carried by ticks, Spencer and Parker ground a few of the creatures in a mortar. They dropped a bit of this material on the skin of a dozen guinea pigs. Half of them got the disease through their unbroken skin! From another group of guinea pigs they shaved patches of fur. On these shaved patches they dropped this soup of death. *All* these guinea pigs got the disease!

Legend of the Valley poured into the schoolhouse. There was the story of the graveyard outside town half filled with spotted fever victims; and the one of the lady past 80 who had lost three husbands to it. And the usual batch of local theories, never to be overlooked. One held that the fever was caused by drinking water which had coursed through sawdust piles at the lumber mills. How, then, explain the fact that the Indians had known this as the poison valley before there were any mills?

As it happened the local theories were valueless. But there was one earlier observation which gave the work a good jumping-off place. In 1906, Dr. Howard Taylor Ricketts, a gigantic intellect even at the age of 35, was vacationing in the Valley. Taking a busman's holiday, he proved that the wood tick, *Dermacentor andersoni* was the creature which spread the disease.

So Spencer wasn't exactly in the dark when he started the arduous job of finding a vaccine; a vaccine which would protect ranchers, herders and woodsmen. The job took nearly five years—and cost three lives. The vaccine was wonderful indeed in areas where infected ticks abounded; in the Bitter Root, in Idaho, in Colorado and elsewhere.

The commodious new lab at Hamilton, built to replace the ancient schoolhouse, now makes enough vaccine each year to treat 150,000 people. In an earlier chapter we noted how Cox had devised a means of using eggs to grow the infective material needed for vaccine.

In places where mild strains of the disease predominate the vaccine apparently gives perfect protection; and it reduces mortality from the violent strains by about 90 per cent. Yet this vaccine isn't the complete answer.

It wouldn't, for example, be worth your while or mine to get vaccinated before going on a camping trip. Chances of our getting the disease are altogether too slim for such a precaution. What was needed was a serum—something to save the lives of people after they had contracted spotted fever. And this gets us around to a personable young man from Flat River, Missouri—Dr. Norman Topping.

Topping, 33, son of a company physician at the lead mines in Southeast Missouri, took medicine at the University of Southern California. After getting his M.D. and serving his internship, he got a job with the National Institute of Health in Washington. This was 1937. He was assigned to work with spotted fever. In working with any disease one can learn a lot reading about the work of others; but he can learn a lot more by doing that work himself. So Topping started over ground that had been covered a dozen times before.

In fields around his home at Bethesda, Maryland, a few miles out of Washington, he ran a line of traps—hoping perhaps he could find this disease in native rabbits, squirrels or field mice. He waded through fields covered with brush, dragging along a white outing flannel flag. Ticks by the hundred hopped on the flag.

Back in the lab Topping dumped his ticks in the cocktail mixer invented by Mr. Fred Waring, the orchestra leader. Waring was thinking in terms of frozen dacquiris, gin fizzes and zombies when he invented his machine; but it turned out to be God's own gift to medical research men. In a few minutes it minces lab material—ticks, for example—into a thick, even soup.

Topping shot this puree of death into guinea pigs. When they became feverish he attached new ticks to their shaved bellies; caging them in place with a bit of wire gauze, shaped like a derby. For a few days these ticks would feast on blood of the sick animal. Then they could pass the disease to other guinea pigs.

All this, of course, wasn't without danger. But Topping had taken elaborate precautions. The glass cubicles where he kept his teams of ticks and guinea pigs were guarded like gangsters at a peace conference. They had to be with that stuff loose on the inside, which was as lethal as a headsman's axe. In the first place there was a barrier of gauze stuck around the inside rim of each cubicle. Theoretically, a tick smitten by wanderlust couldn't get by this. A fine mesh screen covered the top of each cage. As an added precaution each cage sat in a shallow pan of cresol. This poisonous moat should stop any ticks that escaped the other barriers. Then, as a final precaution, there was William: a brown-spotted guinea pig with a face that suggested a minus I.Q. Allowed to run free on the floor, he was bait for any ticks that might escape. As a means of self-defense, Topping had taken a tiny shot of Spencer's vaccine. But he couldn't take a dose large enough to insure complete protection because he was unduly sensitive to it.

So things went: grinding ticks, shooting them into guinea pigs; trying to save their lives with the new sulfa drugs—which didn't work. It was all plodding, routine stuff; then one morning . . .

Topping was walking down the corridor of the Institute. It was two days after the Christmas of 1938. A violent frontal headache began pounding the inside of his skull. Then a chill struck that nearly shook his bones apart. He went across the hall from his lab to tell Dyer—Dr. R. E. Dyer, that is, head of all research with infectious diseases. "Hmmm," said Dyer, "interesting. Better get home. I'll send someone to drive you. Any idea what you've got?" This was an old story to the veteran Dyer. He had seen many sicken, then get well; and others sicken and die.

Topping didn't know. Along with spotted fever, he had worked with typhus, and "Q" fever, recently imported from

Australia. He desperately hoped that it was "Q" fever—hoped for it as you or I might hope for a million dollar legacy. "Q" fever was mild stuff. You were sick for only a few weeks. And Topping had seen what that other, that spotted wrath, could do to people. He had seen the pink spots appear on them, and had heard their howls of delirium as those spots turned purple and grew together. And he had seen death at last mercifully rescue them from their misery. So he hoped hard for "Q" fever.

At home he lay in bed for three days trying to recall every move he had made. His wife Helen watched anxiously. She knew what had happened to Noguchi's assistant, and how the disease had killed Bill Gettinger, Henry Cowan and Roy Kerlee—all of the service. She listened while her husband stated positively that no tick had gotten loose in the lab. Yet he seemed to remember—vaguely—a splash of blood when he was grinding up a batch of them. And he seemed to re-member—also vaguely—a tiny scratch on his hand, gotten while he was emptying an ash pail at home. Possibly . . . Still, he hoped for "Q" fever.

He had been in bed, miserably prostrated for three days, when he looked at his wrist one morning. There were a few innocent-looking blotches of pink! It was spotted fever. An ambulance took him to Walter Reed Hospital.

The siege was long and hard. It would be nice to present the reader with a picture of Topping as the perfect embodiment of scientific detachment; of a man observing first hand the potency of microbes. It would be nice, but it can't be done. Topping was the kind of patient that gives nurses nightmares. People—friends, mind you—came from his own lab to draw blood. They would get Topping's strain of virus started in guinea pigs. He raged at them.

A mouse-like photographer arrived from the Army's medi-cal museum. He wanted to get a picture of a juicy case of spotted fever. Topping threw everything he could lay his hands on. He swore, raged. A nurse made a note on his chart: "Patient very unreasonable." Topping thought he was going to die, and saw absolutely no reason why he should be so damned noble about it.

Dyer shook his head. No, he said, Topping wouldn't die. He had watched others as their heart action faltered; but Topping had plenty of heart left. He would get well.

Dyer was right. He did recover—after a long hospital siege, and weeks spent in the warm Florida sun. Not until March did he get back to the lab; and he was good and mad when he did. Someone *had* to make a serum which would keep people from this wrath; someone had to succeed where the great Noguchi had failed. Topping had a very good idea about who that someone was going to be. He called the animal house and ordered four rabbits.

First he gave them small shots of Spencer's vaccine. Then he began shooting them with highly lethal virus, made from ground up ticks. The vaccine would keep them from dying; and the live virus would make their blood build immunity to the disease—or at least this is what Topping hoped. The thing had been tried before by other workers; but none of them had given rabbits the great hammer blows of virus that Topping proposed to try.

Week after week he ground up ticks, diluted the soup and whirled it in a centrifuge to remove stray legs and wishbones. He squirted larger and larger doses of this almost sure death into rabbits. Some got as much as five whole ticks—enough virus, under ideal circumstances, to give the disease to 75,000 guinea pigs! The fact that they could tolerate so much violence indicated that their blood was swarming with protective factors—antibodies.

Topping began withdrawing this fighting blood—50 cubic centimeters (about two wine glasses) every other week. He allowed the blood to clot and settle, then drew off the straw-colored serum. If the blood held usable protection it would be found in this serum. Finally, he was ready for the test of its efficiency. He called the animal room again. Send up 24 guinea pigs, he said.

Into each of the pigs he shot live virus. Within three days they were feverish. The spotted death was beginning. When this happened Topping divided the animals into two groups of twelve each. One group would be the controls. The other would get the serum he had made.

Each morning as he came into the lab there would be dead guinea pigs among the controls. The others—the ones that got serum—seemed to be sick. But only a few died! This looked good. Topping had taken no great pains to concentrate the serum; to make it as potent as possible. But even in its crude state it *looked* effective. Eleven of the twelve controls eventually died; but there were only three deaths in the serum group!

Next, he tried monkeys. Eight rhesus monks got live virus. All four of the controls died; and all of the four that got serum lived! Never before had monkeys lived after being shot with the Bitter Root strain of virus! This was good. And significant. It was man's turn next.

Topping had been able to accumulate only painfully small amounts of serum. Getting the stuff was tedious, laborious work. In the first place it wasn't safe to draw more than 50 cubic centimeters of blood from a rabbit at one time. By the time this blood serum was sufficiently concentrated for use in man the 50 cubic centimeters shrank 20 times—down to $2\frac{1}{2}$ cubic centimeters. Such a minute amount would be valueless in treating an adult. At least 40 cubic centimeters would be needed—and that represented 16 withdrawals of rabbit blood!

By summer time Topping had enough serum for two patients only. Medically, two such cases would have absolutely no significance. There was always the chance that they would recover without any attention whatsoever. But for his own satisfaction Topping wanted to get the two most miserably ill people he could find.

He saw many cases in and around Washington and discarded those he thought had a 50–50 chance. Finally he found one that suited him; a 5-year-old boy across the Potomac in Alexandria, Virginia. The child's mother remembered that she had picked a tick from his head two weeks before he had gotten sick. The child was in the twelfth day of his illness when Topping saw him; comatose, and covered with a horrid purplish rash. The youngster's doctor conceded that he was as good as dead.

Topping shot a preliminary dose into the child's arm: one cubic centimeter to test for sensitivity to rabbit serum. The reaction was favorable. Then the series began and continued until the child received a total of 20 cubic centimeters. The events that followed weren't dramatic. The child didn't sit up in bed, smile wanly and ask for Mamma as sick children do in the movies. Fever kept at a high level for several days but it was evident that the tide had changed. He was getting better.

Case No. 2 was a 32-year-old woman. A pieced-together case history showed that she had picked ticks off her dog, but so far as was known she hadn't been bitten. (But neither were Spencer's guinea pigs that got the disease through the skin!) She seemed to have virtually no chance of recovery. But her story was much the same as that of the boy: she got 40 cubic centimeters of serum and got well. Again there was no drama—unless we consider it dramatic that she lived.

Topping wasn't unduly elated at either of these recoveries. "They don't mean much," he says. "They might have gotten well anyway." Tests of real significance are under way as this is being written. Advance indications are that they will be successful. If this is so the conquest of this disease, one of the only two ever discovered by Americans, will be completed.

CHAPTER VIII

TROPIC KILLER

Rocky mountain spotted fever is at one end of the scale in point of lives taken. Malaria is at the other. Malaria is Killer No. 1 that silently stalks the warm, damp places of the earth. Microbes of this disease are responsible for a third of all sickness in the tropics. This year they will kill over a million human beings in India. They will account for thousands of lives in Ceylon, and in our own South the death toll will be about 3,000; and malaria will debilitate people so that they are easy prey for other diseases. It will make the muscles of four million people sag; and generally usurp a third of the working time of the Deep South. As a nation we will pay about $500,000,000 tribute to the subtle parasite which produces this great weariness.

Medicine has one principal buttress against this slaughter. It is the miracle drug with a romantic history: quinine. Millions know that their lives depend on it. The unimaginative simply swallow a daily pill to prevent malaria; or gulp great dizzying doses to cure it. Others take it in the form of "gin and tonic water"—seltzer fortified with quinine.

When the poor Southern white notes that his fingernails are turning blue and that he has a teeth-chattering chill, he sends a youngone chasing to the store for a bottle of fever medicine—medicine whose efficacy depends on the quinine it contains.

All these deaths, all this needless suffering and lost labor, understand, take place when quinine is readily available. Anyone can make a guess as to what would happen if the supply were suddenly cut off. The distinct posssibility of this happening is causing a fine case of jitters in the health ministries of most of the world's major countries.

Nearly every ounce of quinine in world trade originates at Java in the Netherlands Indies. Hostile submarines could snip this supply line with a few well-placed torpedoes. In terms of human lives the result of such action would be far more devastating than anything Hitler has been able to accomplish with his complete war.

Quinine is derived from the bark of the cinchona (pronounced (sin-ko'-nah) tree, a native of South America. Long before the white man arrived, Peruvian Indians knew that a bitter tea brewed from this bark would cure malaria. They demonstrated by saving the life of the Countess of Cinchon, wife of the Spanish governor. This word got back to Europe in the 17th century. Not until 1820 did French chemists discover quinine, the life-saving secret held by the bark; and not until 1898 did Sir Ronald Ross of the Indian Medical Service put his finger on the Anopheles mosquito as the sinister night rider that peddled the disease from man to man.

Ross and his successors pieced together the mechanics of spread. They found how a lady Anopheles, who needs blood albumen for her eggs, feasts on a person sick with malaria. Then they went on to discover how the parasites worm their way through the walls of the mosquito stomach, get into the salivary glands, and are spat into the next person bitten. They discovered that the periodic chills which accompany the disease are caused by the liberation of the parasites through the bursting of red blood cells when they can no longer contain their cargo. A single chill represents the liberation of at least 150,000,000 parasites!

While these epochal things were taking place, South American Indians hacked away at forests to provide quinine for the several hundred million people needing it. When it became apparent that the natural supply of cinchona was about to be exhausted, the Dutch sent out an expedition to collect nursery stock. This was in 1854. In 1865, they made a fortunate purchase of cinchona seeds collected by a Britisher living in Puno, Peru. Seeds and nursery stock went to Java, and the Dutch strangle hold on the quinine market became a reality.

With the exception of a small amount of cinchona grown in India and consumed locally, the Dutch have absolute control of the world supply. They strip about 23,000,000 pounds of bark annually from trees grown on 42,000 acres of plantation.

Trees are ready for harvest after ten years' growth. Javanese laborers dig them up and strip bark from trunk, limbs and roots with curved bone knives. Bark is dried, pulverized and mixed with lime and caustic soda. Mineral oil extracts the quinine from this pasty mixture; and acid in turn extracts the drug from the oil. After several more complicated steps pure white crystals of life-saving quinine sulfate result.

The Kina Bureau of Amsterdam, organized in 1913, determines the amount of quinine that will enter world commerce; and allows release of only an amount that will keep world prices stable at around 60 cents per ounce. Export of trees, seeds or nursery stock is absolutely prohibited.

It's a $15,000,000 industry.

What would happen to Southern cotton farmers if quinine were suddenly cut off? No one can say positively, but a reasonable guess gives this picture: with nothing to stop their depredations, malaria parasites would work their way through the blood stream, destroying enough red cells to produce anemia. Many people would die of complete exhaustion. The bodies of others would be too tired to fight off secondary infections. They would perish of such diseases as pneumonia, tuberculosis, dysentery.

Visions of such a series of events have prompted nearly every country in the world which has pretensions to empire to make an effort to crack the Dutch monopoly. Russia has tried to grow cinchona. The French have tried it in Madagascar, the Japanese in Formosa, the British in the Cameroons and the Germans in Tanganyika. Difficulty in procuring hardy root stock and high-yield grafts to apply on them, as well as difficulty in finding the exact climatic conditions required, have combined to thwart these efforts. So far no one has been able to put an appreciable dent in the Dutch monopoly.

The situation has become particularly pressing since the start of the war because malaria can be as terrible as any enemy weapon. During the last World War malaria put 70,000 British soldiers out of the fighting at Salonika; struck down 30,000 in one year in Macedonia, and was similarly devastating in East Africa and Mesopotamia. At one point the situation became particularly difficult. The Dutch threatened to cease cooperating with the Allies. The British rose to the occasion. Either we get quinine, they said in effect, or our navy will see that no one gets it. The Dutch became more tractable.

Malaria is by no means the problem in the United States that it was 50 years ago, when the disease was prevalent in every state east of the Rockies except Maine, New Hampshire and Vermont. Few states had laws requiring doctors to report cases and this allowed statisticians a macabre joke. Year after year they noted that there were more deaths from malaria than cases reported!

Good screening, good drainage and quick isolation of cases —so mosquitoes could not get at them, become infected and pass the disease along—chased the disease south of the Ohio River. But the cotton belt still has an estimated 4,000,000 cases per year. One recent survey, covering 129,000 southern school children, showed parasites in the blood of nearly 6 per cent of them.

Realizing how absolutely essential quinine is to a large part of the United States, federal agencies have been making every possible effort to prepare for a stoppage of supplies. The Health Service recently dispatched a man to South America to check on productive capacity of natural forests. The word he brought back was none too reassuring. Bolivia and Peru produced a minute amount of quinine, he found, but most of their small production was bought up by the Dutch to strengthen their monopoly.

Efforts leading toward a permanent solution are taking place along several lines. In Guatemala several planters, aided by the United States government and one large manufacturing chemist, have spent several years experimenting with the culture of cinchona. There are 40-odd species of this tree and their barks will yield from 1 per cent to 15 per cent quinine. So the problem has been to find the best producers, and the ones which are best adapted to the Guatemalan climate. A great deal of preliminary work with nursery stock has already been done, and plantings on good-sized plots are beginning. As a good-neighbor gesture the federal government has also shipped nursery stock to Brazil.

The United States Department of Agriculture has been working along these same lines in Puerto Rico. Activity centers at the federal experiment station at Mayaguez. Cinchona seedlings grown in Washington are shipped in pots to the Mayaguez station. As many as 3,500 potted seedlings have gone down in one shipment.

After growing for a year or so at the station, they are ready for transplanting. Lacking exact knowledge about the demands of the trees—they seem to like high altitude, tropical sun, and ample rainfall—plantings have been made at various elevations: 1,000, 2,500 and 3,000 feet.

Particular emphasis has been placed on culture in the Maricao Insular Forest. While the Department of Agriculture hopes that local capital will become interested in large scale plantation culture, they don't want to bank too heavily on this. Hence the forest plantings. A good stand of trees growing under natural conditions would represent an excellent reserve of vital quinine, which could be drawn upon in times of national emergency.

Research men in Washington are likewise making an effort to save the situation. By a curious coincidence six chemists working for the National Institute of Health began looking for new quinine substitutes the day war began.

At the start they realized that it would be virtually impossible to make quinine synthetically. The molecule is large and incredibly complex. To reconstruct it, borrowing atoms of carbon, hydrogen, oxygen and nitrogen from readily available chemicals might be possible; but the steps required would almost surely make the process prohibitively expensive. Somewhere within this giant molecule, they felt, was hidden the active principle—the malaria-killing principle. Their efforts have been directed toward finding this magic.

French chemists tried the same thing. After synthesizing over 700 new substances—any one of which would fit in the quinine molecule—they gave up the job. The Germans had more luck. They produced two antimalarial drugs, plasmochin and atebrin. These drugs are effective and tremendously valuable, but they have two big drawbacks. They are expensive and they require medical supervision. These two things put them out of the reach of a large proportion of the millions who have malaria, which is primarily a poor man's disease.

There are many reasons for this somewhat frenzied activity, apart from the fact that 14,000,000 people in the Southeastern United States live constantly with malaria at their doorsteps. It is quite possible for the disease again to spread into regions where it has been barred for decades. Malaria mosquitoes are prevalent in most states. A nibble at a person sick with the disease starts the chain going. Sporadic outbreaks occasionally occur in the North but are quickly squelched with the aid of quinine. The one a few years ago at Camden, New Jersey, will illustrate.

Cases began to occur in a most unlikely place; in a suburb recently built for well-to-do people. A shrewd epidemiologist quickly put his finger on the cause. Mosquitoes by the millions were breeding in decorative ponds and pools. All they needed to touch off an epidemic was a source of blood parasites. These were finally furnished by a malaria carrier, a visitor from Costa Rica.

Another factor worrying the Health Service is the fact that strains of violent malaria are loose within easy plane range of the United States. Brazil has such a killer, spread by the *Anopheles gambiae.* This mosquito was brought across the South Atlantic by planes from Africa. This insect has already killed ten per cent of the people in some districts and a heroic effort is under way to exterminate it—history's first example of such a gigantic undertaking.

A similar malaria is rampant along the Burma Road which the Chinese constructed as a supply route to the outside world. Several times this epidemic malaria stopped road construction as coolies fled in terror from "black-water fever"— the violent malaria in which the microbes explode blood cells.

Preventive work is proceeding in the Southern United States. WPA projects have drained nearly three million acres of swamp and applied two million gallons of spray. Tens of thousands of houses have been screened. The work has helped the situation but has by no means eliminated the Killer No. 1 of the tropics. As long as there are men with malaria to furnish blood meals to mosquitoes, the disease will be with us. There remains but one thoroughly tested means of controlling this situation, and that means is quinine. It is going to be difficult to break the tight monopolistic hold which the Dutch have on this drug. But we are trying.

CHAPTER IX

THE MAGIC ISLANDS

As we review the recent accomplishments of the research laboratory a question naturally arises. What else is there to do? What remains in the file of medicine's unfinished business? Unhappily, there are thousands of jobs awaiting the agile mind. Most research men are frank to admit that the cream has been skimmed. The easy jobs have been done. From now on it will grow increasingly difficult. The present status of work with diabetes offers a good illustration.

The laboratory where the greater part of all diabetes research has taken place is a curious one. It has no Hollywood touches: no glistening gadgets, no mystifying machines. Quite the reverse. Everything is on the grubby side. The work tables are scarred with age and eaten with acids. There is an ancient fume cupboard to carry away lung-biting gases; and the usual disorderly mass of technical glassware. Nothing, you agree, to suggest that you are standing on some of the holiest ground in the world of medical research. A modest bronze plaque, hung high enough on the wall to escape notice, explains:

". . . In May, 1921, Frederick Grant Banting and Charles Herbert Best, both graduates of the University of Toronto, conducted in this room the experiments which culminated in the discovery of insulin."

That was a heroic piece of work. The lives of nearly half a million U.S. diabetics rest on it. Two million more people now living will contract diabetes before they die—and will need this colorless fluid magic. It has bestowed on human beings the richest of all gifts—life itself. Diabetic children have won an additional 30 years; and life expectancy of middle-aged groups has been extended twelve years!

Reflect on these things and wonder why, in heaven's name, this lab hasn't been placed in honorary retirement; protected perhaps by a velvet rope. Yet it is just as well that it didn't win these dubious honors. Work just completed in this shabby, cluttered little hole in the wall holds enormous promise for millions not yet born. The original discovery of insulin gave life and hope to people facing certain doom. This new work presents experimental evidence that diabetes can be prevented; that generations to come may escape the lethal fury of this debilitating sickness!

Presently, we'll see the exciting details of the work which led to this conclusion. Meanwhile, let's understand the mechanics of diabetes. Man's pancreas, shaped like a pollywog, lies just back of the stomach. It serves a dual function. It secretes a daily pint and a half of digestive fluid which it pours into the small intestine. More vital, the gland secretes minute quantities of another substance which it empties directly into the blood stream. This is the hormone insulin.

Insulin is manufactured by tiny "island" cells, each independent of the other. The average pancreas, small organ though it is, contains from 750,000 to a million and a quarter of these islet cells. The insulin they secrete governs the body's utilization of sugar. When adequate insulin is present sugar is burned rapidly into energy. When it isn't, the body burns stored fats and proteins. The body wastes away and the sufferer lives constantly with an unquenchable thirst, an unappeasable hunger. Poisonous matter resulting from the combustion of fats accumulates in the blood. So does unburned sugar. If the condition goes unattended—if insulin isn't given by hypodermic—coma and death follow.

Insulin, the magic which allows diabetics to live more or less comfortably with this fright of a disease, was discovered by a two-man team: Charles H. Best, a medical student whose education was interrupted by war service in the British tank corps;

Frederick G. Banting, a surgeon who dropped a rural practice to follow a brilliant research hunch. Banting died tragically in the crash of a Britain-bound bomber.

Banting and Best found how to extract insulin from beef pancreas (sweetbread); and discovered that this animal organ supplied enough insulin to keep the average diabetic going for twenty days. Scheduled shots—as many as four a day—gave years of useful life to such people as the late King George V of England, George Eastman, H. G. Wells, Hugh Walpole and hundreds of thousands of other less famed diabetics. It was discovered barely in time to give Dr. George R. Minot the new lease on life he needed to go on and discover the liver treatment for an equally fatal disease—pernicious anemia.

But the finding of insulin wasn't the end. From the research man's point of view it was the bare beginning. No one knew why the island cells, discovered by and named for the German pathologist Paul Langerhans, suddenly ceased functioning. In other words no one knew what. *caused* diabetes. Insulin, of course, wouldn't cure the disease. And there was no means of prevention. So there were quantities of work to be done with this sickness which converted active, robust people into wretched bags of bones.

Unnoticed and unpublicized, work continued throughout the world. Enormous strides were taken during depression years. Like clues in a mystery, fragments began to fit together to make a significant picture.

Herbert McLean Evans, great University of California biologist, stumbled on a startling fact. He was studying the growth-promoting factors in the pituitary, the body's master gland. Repeatedly he shot dogs with extracts taken from the anterior portion of this gland. By chance, he happened to note that the animals became diabetic! Why this senseless fact? No one knew.

Then Bernardo Houssay, South American researcher, hit upon another fact which moved all diabetes research along another notch. Everyone knew that if the pancreas were removed from a dog, that dog would die within a fortnight. Houssay discovered that if the pituitary were also removed the dog would live indefinitely!

From here it was a natural step to London—and the work of Frank Young, a former student of Best's at the University of Toronto. This big, taciturn researcher, working at Britain's National Institute of Medical Research, found that if, for the period of a few weeks dogs got daily shots of pituitary a permanent diabetes developed. Here was the basis for a good guess as to the cause of this wasting sickness. *Perhaps*—the italics are important—it was caused by a too active pituitary. This gland secreted a stimulating juice which literally worked the islet cells of the pancreas to death.

Here we swing back to Toronto, home port of diabetes research, and a yellow brick building, blackened by the coal soot of dozens of bitter winters. This is the Medical Building on the University campus, scene of Banting and Best's original work. It was here that a trio of top-notch research men began wrangling with the problem of diabetes prevention. The men: James Campbell, young Scotch-born bio-chemist; Reginald Haist, also young, also somewhat grimly intent on whipping this thing; Charles Best, who seems altogether too boyish, too apple-cheeked, for his position as a medical immortal.

The trio sized up their problem. Evans and Houssay had produced convincing evidence that pituitary extract would produce diabetes; and Young had indicated why. Very well. Was there anything which would counteract this effect? Anything which would, perhaps, let these cells which were being worked to death rest for a while, and regenerate their strength? If such a thing could be found it would be of incalculable benefit. It might mean that the 27 out of every 1,000 girl babies born this year would escape the diabetic death forecast for them by statisticians. It would mean new hope for whole generations to come.

Diet represented a logical point of attack. As long ago as 1914 Dr. Frederick M. Allen, then working at the Rockefeller Institute, had indicated the profound effect diet has on diabetes. He had outlined the starvation diets which made pitiable runts out of children, and bony invalids out of adults. These individuals paid terrible prices for the few additional years of life they gained. But Allen's ideas represented the logical jumping off place for the new work.

Rats were selected as the animals for these new researches. Dozens of them were ordered down from the attic animal room—where low beams and door frames are fiendishly set to scalp the unwary. These docile creatures were required to answer one question puzzling the experimentors: could carefully concocted diets remove part of the load from the pancreas and if so, how much of that load?

The rats were divided into three groups. One got a normal diet; the second fasted; the third subsisted largely on fats—which require little insulin for utilization. After a week of this the animals were killed, their pancreases removed. Assays indicated that the pancreases of the fasting, and of the fat-fed animals contained only half as much insulin as the controls!

Significance? It looked as if starvation in one case, and fat feeding in the other had allowed the pancreas to go on a half-time schedule. Here was a means of giving an overworked organ a rest cure! Rest could work wonders with injured bones, damaged lung tissue, or overburdened hearts. Would rest do as much for the microscopic islet cells that had been going at too fast a clip? More work had to be done before this one could be answered.

Next step was to see if periodic shots of insulin would lower the pancreas's content of this natural secretion. It did. Here, then, was a second way to let this gland rest. Up to this point Haist, Campbell and Best had worked with healthy animals. They had built up a body of convincing evidence that diet and insulin would allow the pancreas to drowse along on half time.

But they hadn't come to grips with the big problem. Now they were ready for it. Let's set the problem up.

Experimental work with dogs had showed the link between diabetes and an overactive pituitary. Very likely the same picture held with man; autopsies frequently revealing widespread damage to the islet cells. Now the question arose: was there anything which would offset the destructive effect of pituitary substance?

Insulin appeared as a likely contender. Simultaneously the researchers shot a group of dogs with two brews: destructive pituitary, healing insulin. Day after day the creatures got the two gland juices. And day after day the two scientific cubs checked blood and urine of the animals for telltale rises in sugar. But the sugar stayed resolutely at normal! It wasn't accumulating in the blood, or being discarded by the kidneys in poisonous, sickening quantities! Insulin, it appeared, had worked prophylactically. It had prevented the disease which should have occurred with doleful regularity.

As a further check, they would have to investigate the islet cells themselves. Haist, working with a colleague, Dr. Arthur Ham, began anesthetizing dogs. Deftly he shaved away a little belly hair, made an incision and snipped out a bit of pancreas. This fragment was treated with paraffin to make it rigid, then cut into thin slivers by the lab's version of the restaurant bread slicer. There was rejoicing at what the eye saw when these slivers were viewed through the microscope! There was none of the watery bloat that marks an islet cell bound for destruction. They were well, healthy, normal!

One more check was required to complete the work. Two dogs were selected for this experiment. For 30 days each animal got a daily shot of pituitary. One ate a normal diet, one subsisted largely on fat. The one on a normal diet became permanently diabetic; the other recovered. Here, then, was additional evidence that the destructive work of the pituitary could be overcome.

All this sounds quite easy and simple—on paper. But months of drudgery were required: snipping pancreases out of rats and dogs; extracting the insulin; shooting it into mice and noting how much was needed to send them into convulsions. Only in this way—a single assay might require 250 mice—was it possible to determine the amount of insulin an exercised pancreas contained.

To sum up accomplishments, the researchers had found two methods of resting islet cells possibly bound for exhaustion; and two methods of combatting a too active pituitary.

Translation of this work to man shouldn't be too difficult. Clinical work has already started in several places. People predisposed to diabetes by heredity are periodically tested for telltale rises in blood and urine sugar. Immediately they occur, the patient has to modify his diet. Fats—cream, butter, bacon —will, for a while, have to supply the calories usually supplied by sweets. This will rest islet cells. An occasional small shot of insulin must be given to combat the harmful effects of too much pituitary.

A few figures will indicate why the clinical work now going forward should be prayerfully attended. Despite the achievement of Banting and Best in discovering insulin, death rates from diabetes continue to mount. Today 30,000 people die of this disease in the United States each year. Why this shocking number? There are several explanations. Overeating has become more general—and 80 per cent of all diabetics are overweight. Better diagnostic methods now detect the disease where, at an earlier date, it escaped notice. And, on top of these factors, there is an accumulation of diabetic patients who are just beginning to die, but would have died years earlier had it not been for insulin. This magic stuff can't confer immortality.

These points help explain the rise in diabetic deaths; but have done nothing to stop the upsurge. We can't persuade a nation to diet; and can't escape heredity factors by forcing women from diabetic families to marry men from families free of it. So the problem has grown; diabetes achieving a greater importance for some age groups than tuberculosis.

Because of these considerations it has become increasingly urgent for some research man to find a means of prevention; a procedure which would ward off this terrible sickness as vaccine wards off smallpox. The new work at the University of Toronto appears to have laid the groundwork for such a tremendous accomplishment.

For his part Dr. Best likes to emphasize one point. The present work holds no promise whatsoever of *curing* old cases of the disease. To point up its preventive potentialities he would like to see a wide-scale clinical test, of the type dear to the hearts of all research men. He would like to have a group of 500 children predisposed to diabetes by heredity. Half would get treatment to rest the pancreas, half would go without it. He realizes that "many years may be required to complete the obvious extension of the present experiments . . . but sufficient information is now available to show that production of diabetes in experimental animals . . . may be prevented . . ."

CHAPTER X

WEARY WORLD

THE whole question of fatigue represents another piece of unfinished business. Human beings are a weary lot. They are tired from tennis, golf, wood-chopping, plowing. Anything we do—if we do it long enough—makes us tired. Muscles get saggy and bed becomes surpassingly beautiful.

Until a few years ago the biologist had an engagingly simple picture of this feeling which causes half the grief and bad temper in a drowsy world. All due to accumulated lactic acid in muscle tissue, he said. He even had proof.

The classic experiment ran this way: first the biologist would snip a leg muscle out of a frog or rat. He'd immerse the muscle in cool salted water and hang a weight on one end of it. Then he'd stimulate it with electricity so that it would contract, lifting the weight. This would continue until the muscle was exhausted and could work no more. Routine chemical analysis invariably showed a large increase in lactic acid—the same stuff that contributes to the sour taste in buttermilk.

Other research men took up here. They withdrew blood from runners before and after dashes, checked it, and noted increased lactic acid. This seemed to seal the case. Then other checks unsealed it. Field hands, miserably weary from a day's cotton hoeing, showed no appreciable lactic acid increase! The same thing held for other men who had done long sustained labor. Too bad, concluded the researchers. It had looked so easy.

Things stood in this muddled condition when, in 1927, Harvard set up its Fatigue Laboratory. Chemists, biologists and physiologists were tucked off in a corner of the basement of Morgan Hall, one of the group of Boston buildings that make up the University's Graduate School of Business Administration. The tie-up between business and fatigue seems odd; but fatigue is a far greater industrial problem than tariffs, labor unions or murderous competition.

The laboratory where these men work is fatiguing to behold. It contains every conceivable piece of machinery to give living creatures the droops. There are treadmills for rats and dogs, stationary bicycles and rowing machines for men, heat chambers to bring on the lassitude experienced in the tropics, and sealed chambers to duplicate the conditions that wear down mountain climbers.

Object of all this is to make a subject as tired as possible, as quickly as possible. Then try to detect what has happened to his body chemistry. To this end young men work themselves to a lather on rowing machines, and old men (one subject was 91 years old) jog wearily along on treadmills. Attendants collect air expired by laboring lungs, and blood samples for chemical analysis.

Classic story of the laboratory concerns a visiting Englishman who wandered in one day and was mistaken for a volunteer subject. While he protested through his whiskers, one attendant strapped a mask over his face and another pushed him on a fast-moving treadmill. He was removed after a few minutes and stretched, panting, on a bed while an attendant punctured his ear lobe for a blood withdrawal. Before fainting he muttered something that sounded like "crazy Americans."

Scores of famous athletes have worked on the Harvard treadmill; such men as Archie San Romani, Don Lash and Glenn Cunningham. Barry Wood, All-America Harvard footballer, also worked in the laboratory and even contributed a paper to scientific literature while still a premedical student. Wood was interested in the increase in white blood cells (leucocytes) after sustained labor and used to wheedle blood donations from football players before and after hard games.

As a result of all this work, the Harvard researchers have built up a comprehensive picture of fatigue. They recognize the fact that as a word fatigue is about as vague as beauty— which covers everything from the saucer-lipped ladies of Africa to the cuties of Hollywood. But they are getting order out of this confusion. They know that the tiredness felt by a dash runner is distinct from that felt by a factory worker and stems from different chemical processes. They also recognize the fact that much weariness traces to boredom and hence is a problem for the psychologist, rather than the bio-chemist.

By and large, the laboratory workers—principally Drs. David Bruce Dill, John W. Thompson, W. H. Forbes and Robert E. Johnson—have chosen to look on fatigue in terms of adaptation. A well-trained stevedore can toss freight all day and a woman can shop for hats without suffering any undue discomfort. But let them change places and they would be fagged out in a short time. The point is that neither is adapted to the work of the other.

Given enough time, man can accommodate himself to almost any conditions. He lives everywhere. He has permanent settlements in towns that frequently have winter temperatures of 50 below zero, and in deserts with sun temperature of 150 degrees and higher. In one experiment two British scientists put a man in a chamber heated with dry air to a temperature of 250 degrees F.! He remained there for fifteen minutes and suffered no particular damage. The man's adaptive body had generated quantities of perspiration and evaporation of this fluid had kept his body cool within safe limits.

The Harvard men set up their case. Since fatigue seemed to be very largely a question of adaptation, why not study men as they adapted themselves to conditions as dramatic as possible? See what happened to them, and try to shed new light on the chemistry of tiredness?

Pursuing this course, they have gone on expeditions to the flaming hot Black Canyon region of the Colorado River basin; and into the sweltering tropical humidity of Barro Colorado Island in the Panama Canal's Gatun Lake. They have worked in the Youngstown steel mills and in the highest permanent town in the world, a sulphur mining camp perched 17,500 feet up on Mt. Aucanquilcha in Chile.

The Harvard men have brought back quantities of practical information. The trip to Boulder City, Nevada, site of the Boulder Dam construction camp, will illustrate. During the first year of construction in this sweltering rock crevice, fifteen men died of heat, and scores of others had heat cramps—a malady accompanied by pains comparable only to those of childbirth.

It had been previously suggested that heat cramps and heat fatigue might trace to loss of body salt by excessive sweating. Under really severe conditions a man loses as much as four gallons of moisture a day. Taking this as a cue the Harvard men began investigating that most un-Harvard substance—sweat.

For hours on end workers walked on treadmills, clothed only in socks and shorts. Weighings before and after indicated the amount of sweat that had been lost; and baths in rubber tubs filled with distilled water showed composition of that sweat. An alarming loss of body salt was indicated. This was particularly true for newcomers. Men long on the job sweated just as much but their sweat contained less salt. It was the old business of adaptation. After a while their bodies had learned to conserve salt.

Once large-scale tests had indicated the extent of salt loss it was a simple matter to remedy this deficiency: by adding salt to drinking water. After this was done workmen remained alert and fresh when they otherwise would have been miserably tired. Heat deaths stopped and heat cramps became rare. A similar piece of work in Youngstown steel mills ended with equally striking results.

As a consequence of this work, salt in drinking water is now routine in hot industries; in glass-making, steel, baking and even on the Detroit assembly lines when a heat wave strikes. Astute football trainers feed salt—or bouillon, which is more palatable—to players in hot, early-season games. For the first time in years, the Duke University team, which adopted the practice in 1938, went through a season without a single case of heat cramps.

Oxygen starvation contributes to another type of fatigue— the panting tiredness felt after hill climbing or other sustained hard work. Study of this phenomenon took the Harvard group to the Andean sulphur camp already mentioned. Lured by high wages, workmen live in bleak stone huts perched at an altitude at which no vegetable life exists. Newcomers always have violent headaches, and nausea, and may even lose consciousness. Yet such is the body's adaptability that native workmen even play football; a slow-motion variety to be sure, but football just the same.

They erroneously attribute their ability to work in this spot on the roof of the world to the fact that they constantly chew dried cocoa leaves dipped in ash. From this they extract minute amounts of cocaine. A better explanation of their work ability is that they have an abnormally large number of red blood cells to carry oxygen. Infants, however, do not have this faculty.

Women must go to lower altitudes to deliver their babies. The air at the camp is so thin—one breath will deliver only half as much oxygen as a similar breath at sea level—that newborn infants are suffocated.

Working here and in a temporary camp on the mountain summit (20,140 feet) the Harvard men underwent considerable hardship. One man lost 26 pounds and the average weight loss was 15 pounds. Thawing canned food in water which boiled at 175 degrees F. instead of at 212 was a tedious process. Six or seven rapid steps left them breathless and their lips were always blue from oxygen starvation.

Study of blood samples withdrawn at this altitude explained the weariness that comes with being "winded." During a heavy expenditure of energy the body burns fat and sugar rapidly. It must have oxygen for this process. Failure of lungs and circulatory system to supply it results in fatigue.

The blood of the well-trained athlete has greater oxygen-carrying capacity than the blood of an untrained man; and the athlete's tissue can absorb oxygen faster. This explains why Tarzan Weissmuller easily swims distances that would leave most of us as breathless as a beached flounder.

Treadmill measurements show a man's total capacity for work and the efficiency with which he does that work. Note in passing that man is nowhere like the perfect machine high-school biology teachers would have us believe him to be. The Diesel engine, the high-compression auto motor and the mercury vapor turbine all surpass him. Man's efficiency ranges from 16 to 20 per cent—which is to say that only this amount of chemical energy consumed as food is converted into external mechanical energy. A consoling thought for the middle-aged: At 50 a man's body may be far more efficient than it was at 20.

Figures so far available disclose that a man can expend energy at the rate of one third of his capacity without becoming unduly tired. Any factory management that was so minded could check any employee against the requirements of his job to see whether he was safely inside this limit.

The laboratory workers have yet to produce a magic pill that will banish fatigue. Much work must be done before the tired feeling that catches up with us at least once a day can be completely explained away. But a systematic start has been made. They have discovered how salt-replacement can offset weariness in hot industries; and how energy expenditure limits should be set for all factories. Other facts will accrue as they penetrate the maze that surrounds the chemistry of weariness.

CHAPTER XI

LIFE FOR SALE

THE work of medical research men would, for the most part, be valueless if it weren't for the large manufacturers of drugs and biological products. These people put new discoveries on drugstore shelves where doctors can get at them. Instead of making vaccine by the cubic centimeter, they make it by the barrel; instead of saving the lives of mice, they save the lives of men.

By and large, these manufacturers are doing an excellent job. They are subsidizing university research and carrying on large programs of their own. All this work is aimed at providing us with better, cheaper drugs and biologicals to cure our sicknesses. In this chapter we will look at Lederle Laboratories. Lederle is chosen chiefly because it is one of the most active companies in the research field. Its big establishment at Pearl River, N.Y. looks more like a farm than a manufacturing plant.

Five hundred horses live in miraculously sanitary stalls and calves romp in well-tailored fields. Two thousand hogs live in pens as clean as hog pens can be, and 10,000 rabbits live in spray-cooled hutches. There are dogs, chickens and other animals to complete the barnyard scene. These animals are used to make serums, vaccines and antitoxins which prevent death at the hands of pneumonia, diphtheria, smallpox and a host of other diseases.

Follow a horse through his residence at the farm; a horse assigned to making the antitoxin which prevents jaws locking with tetanus. This stuff neutralizes the toxin—poison—that microbes discharge in open wounds.

Our horse is no beauty. Perhaps he has lop ears and a sway back. Very likely he has some foot ailment that lost him his job pulling a milk wagon. But looks won't matter to the mother whose child needs protection when a rusty nail or an exploding firecracker lodge tetanus spores deep under the skin.

Outside the horse's stall hangs a temperature chart. He eats the choicest foods and has spacious paddocks for exercise. For these considerations he must submit to a tiny shot of tetanus toxoid. Week after week injections increase in size as the animal's blood builds tolerance. After a while the horse is hyper-immune. With ease, he can withstand great lethal jolts of the microbe which a few months earlier would have killed him swiftly and surely. His blood is filled with protective factors to save lives of motor accident victims, soldiers, and others.

Fortnightly withdrawals of this precious blood begin: blood to be processed into antitoxin. Life for the horse is rich, easy and humdrum so long as protection holds up. When it drops he gives way to another animal.

Founding of Lederle dates back to 1906. That year Dr. William Hallock Park, of the New York Health Department, was busy with one of history's most glowing medical crusades: the one against diphtheria. This disease was snuffing out lives of 2,500 New York City children each year, and was similarly ravaging the rest of the country. In Germany, Emil von Behring had discovered the means of using horses to make antitoxin—antitoxin which kept the death grip of diphtheria from the throats of children.

Park got quantities of this material manufactured and prodded doctors into using it. Complaints came from all sides. This horse serum made children deathly ill. Why, said some, the serum sickness was as bad as diphtheria itself. The complaints were legitimate so Park hired a chemist and set him to work. Manufacture of the purified antitoxin he produced began in the city's laboratories. But no commercial maker of biological products was disposed to adopt the expensive process so the rest of the country could benefit.

Park, the crusader, marched to the health commissioner, the late Ernst J. Lederle. If the country's children were to be saved from the criminal assaults of diphtheria someone had to market this new antitoxin. *Had* to, Park said.

Lederle tugged his long moustache, thought a while, and finally announced a decision. He would raise funds to finance the venture. Lederle Laboratories moved into an ancient brownstone house on upper Fifth Avenue. In its better days it had been a boarding house. A dozen workers began drawing blood from horses in a nearby livery stable; and extra quantities arrived in ice-packed milk cans from a farm in the suburbs. Stanley D. Beard took charge of manufacturing and research—a post he still holds.

Lederle remained an independent until 1930 when it was integrated into the huge American Cyanamid Company. Today it sprawls over a 200-acre farm. There are 65 buildings. As in the case of a munitions plant, especially violent things are segregated from other activity. There is one building for making smallpox vaccine. Gas gangrene, the soldier killer, has another. Virus research is carried on in a building to which no outsider is admitted. All tetanus work is done well off in a corner of the property.

Pigs used to make protection against hog cholera (more of this is sold than any other biological product) have no traffic with rabbits which produce pneumonia serum. Dogs making rabies vaccine never see sheep, cattle, pigeons and chickens assigned to other jobs.

Research plays a dominant rôle in this vast plant. Other industries may survive without such investigative effort, but for the manufacturer of biological and pharmaceutical products, research represents the sole means of expansion. Markets for existing products have been thoroughly explored. Only when new or better ones are found to save us the drudgery of sickness and the penalty of death can payrolls be enlarged.

Let the work of Dr. Ivan Parfentjev illustrate. Parfentjev, a big, baldish Russian émigré was working at Duke University in 1935 under a Lederle grant. He asked that a specific project be assigned him. The company sent along a few cubic centimeters of diphtheria antitoxin, requesting that he attempt an extra refining step.

There were, his instructions said in effect, many inactive things in the product. Park's chemist had removed some of this material but in the 30 years that followed no one had been able to radically improve his technique. Cases of serum sickness still occurred, adding this burden to children already sick with diphtheria.

No one felt that Parfentjev would succeed. Some of the world's greatest chemists had broken heads against this problem without result. But it was worth a chance. Longshot players are more plentiful in this profession than they are at the race tracks.

The Russian set to work. At the start he realized that the troublesome factors in the antitoxin were probably proteins. He reasoned his way through another step. Pepsin is the digestive juice that dissolves protein in animal and human stomachs. Very well, why not try and digest the protein out of the antitoxin with pepsin taken from the stomach of a hog? Easy enough, so far. But there was a stumbling block. Pepsin had to do its work in the presence of acid—and acid would kill the active principle of the antitoxin.

Parfentjev jiggled his solutions and threaded his way between two unyielding facts: acid weak enough not to hurt the antitoxin, and pepsin in sufficient concentration to gobble up protein. His lab lights burned long past bedtime for the rest of the Duke campus. After a few months he sent a few vials of miraculously clear antitoxin to the Pearl River plant. He followed, with his baggage—by invitation. He had reduced volume 40 per cent without impairing potency! His method was immediately adapted to make better weapons to fight tetanus, scarlet fever, gas gangrene, and staphylococcus infections. His antitoxins cut serum sickness 50 per cent. Another story is similarly heartening: the story of pernicious anemia . . .

This ghoulish disease occurs when the body forgets how to make red blood cells. Tissue starvation and death are the end results. In 1926, Drs. George Minot and William Murphy of Boston, and George Whipple of Rochester made the epochal discovery which won them a Nobel Prize. Liver, they found, when consumed in sufficient quantities would ward off death. But patients had to eat great gagging quantities. The diet became a torture worthy of the ancient Chinese. Ground liver fed by a stomach tube and a nauseous powdered extract which had to be taken three or four times a day offered little help.

Scientists undertook making a material pure enough for injection. Dr. Guy Clark, a Lederle chemist with wise, owlish eyes, was one of these workers. For months his laboratory gave off the sickening, sweetish stench of cooking liver. He ground organs from hogs, calves and cows, extracted vital components with weak acids and took off fractions. Finally he turned up with a juice which pleased him. There was but one way to test its value. Man is the only experimental animal for pernicious anemia research.

Three cubic centimeter doses of this potent stuff went into the hip muscles of a patient. Results were highly promising but a certain amount of pain attended the injection. Clark worked three more years purifying the extract; finally got it down to one cubic centimeter. These minute shots each represent a quarter pound of liver put directly into the circulatory system where it is needed—enough to last from one to three weeks. Tens of thousands of patients began receiving this painless magic and Lederle began buying liver in dozen carload lots.

Rabbit serum for pneumonia represents another recent research triumph. Original work which led to use of this animal was started by Lederle, and the Rockefeller Institute demonstrated the efficacy of such serum. Rabbit advantages include ease and speed in preparing serum. Where it takes two years to bring a horse up to a maximum production, a rabbit achieves this in eight weeks.

There are other advantages as well. No manufacturers could afford to keep refreshing stocks of perishable serum for the rarely occurring pneumonias. Types 27, 30, 32, for example, did not present themselves frequently enough to merit keeping horses in serum production. Cheapness of the rabbit made it possible to stock sera for all 32 types of pneumonia—including Type 3, most lethal of the lot for which horse serum was never effective. Use of this weapon in conjunction with the new drug sulfapyridine is saving a large proportion of the hundred thousand lives formerly taken annually by pneumonia.

The vast Lederle plant markets a bewildering array of products: sulfapyridine to fight off bacterial diseases, serums, vaccines, antitoxins—for man, cattle, dogs and hens. There are shots to make measles mild and whopping cough whoopless; and protein extracts to overcome sensitivity to shad roe, Swiss chard and tapioca.

People are allergic to proteins hidden in dusts, pollens, foods. To combat this doctors inoculate them with ever-mounting doses of the protein causing trouble. The body builds resistance to overcome sensitivity. Lederle stocks hundreds of extracts for this purpose.

At vegetable markets it buys crates of endive, dandelion and dill. Fish and meat stores provide fluke and flounder, venison and veal. Professional collectors gather pollen from ragweed and various grasses. Proteins extracted from these things with saline solution are refined and bottled. But before it goes on the market each batch must be tested on sensitive individuals. Lederle has a long list of these unfortunates; people who have allergies ranging from duck feathers to Jerusalem artichokes.

An amazing variety of products enter the plant to be processed, standardized and marketed. An affiliated company sends vitamins and new synthetic drugs like sulfanilamide. Dried leaves from the wildflower foxglove arrive to be converted into digitalis which will save failing hearts. The war having radically reduced German and British supplies, WPA workers are now investigating possibilities of commercial culture.

The company maintains a special collection service to gather placentas in New York maternity hospitals. These placentas are converted into a product to modify measles; make it a mild disease of short duration, rather than a serious, frequently fatal malady. A striking story lies behind this effort. Observers long ago noted that for the first few months of life infants are immune to most childhood diseases. They get this protection from their mothers' blood. Protection wears off when an infant starts manufacturing its own supply.

Since afterbirth tissue is rich in maternal blood, Lederle began collecting this material. A few cubic centimeters of serum from this source give older children the natural protection that infants have.

Research at Lederle has paid off handsomely. During depression years employment tripled. In the past five years sales have doubled and redoubled. Facts like these explain why the company is expending nearly half a million dollars a year on 69 research projects in its own plant and 30 others in various universities.

Altruism has no part in motivating expenditures on this scale. That this work might save thousands of lives is purely incidental. Lederle, like an ever-increasing number of wise companies, has simply recognized that research is destined to play an increasingly important rôle in all industry. And having recognized this, it has gone into the business wholeheartedly.

CHAPTER XII

BEGINNING OF LIFE

Dr. Couney was horrified by a wastage of human life that he observed. It wasn't a wastage caused by microbes; but wastage of a very special sort. He set out to correct it and has spent 45 years on the job. Possibly he doesn't belong here in the company of Felton, Doisy and Domagk; yet, by and large, the aims of all four men are parallel. They wish to save human life.

Dr. Martin Arthur Couney, 72, has the gentle, fatherly manner of a God-fearing German burgher. He operates hospitals that are utterly unique; hospitals where visitors pay 25 cents to gape at patients. Funds thus collected have gone to provide free care for more than 8,000 very special infants —those born prematurely into the world.

Sickness, overwork, bad diet or nerves can cause a mother to prematurely project an infant into the world for which it is unprepared. When this happens in the fifth month the infant may live as long as 48 hours but it dies in the end. Vital organs fail to function. In the sixth month there is a chance. Dr. Couney has made a life work of giving infants that chance.

Something like ten million people have paid to see the first faltering steps of life in Couney's incubators; people in Berlin, Paris, London, Atlantic City and Coney Island; at the Century of Progress in Chicago and at the World's Fair in New York. What they have seen is an odd admixture of showmanship and philanthropy.

Dr. Couney insists that he does not exhibit babies. He exhibits his *system* of keeping the feeble flame of life burning in infants that have weighed as little as a pound and a half. Couney has received the endorsement of such people as Dr. Julius Hess, great Chicago pediatrician, Morris Fishbein of the American Medical Association, and of a number of medical and public health organizations. This recognition is based on results achieved: 80 per cent of his babies have survived, whereas 50 per cent would be a highly acceptable figure.

The system consists of providing superb nursing care; and duplicating so far as possible conditions of the womb in the outside world. This means a constant supply of nourishing food, warmth and an extra supply of oxygen. Perhaps the best way to observe the Couney technique is to follow an infant through its course.

Baby R. was born two-and-a-half months prematurely, weighing three pounds, two ounces. The obstetrician was completely frank with the father. The infant, he said, had virtually no chance of survival. Its lungs had failed to inflate properly and it was blue from oxygen starvation.

To care for it at the hospital would be crushingly expensive. The baby would need three shifts of nurses a day for perhaps two months. There would be added costs of incubator, oxygen, medical care, and mother's milk. The bill would perhaps run to $5,000. And quite frankly, he added, the hospital didn't offer facilities comparable to those offered by the Midway attraction at Coney Island operated by Dr. Couney. In this unique hospital, the doctor explained, the baby would pay for its keep by allowing others to watch the drama of a life being saved. There would be no cost whatsoever. The father grasped at this opportunity.

A telephone call summoned a singular ambulance. Its engine was slung low so radiator water would rise to heat a tiny cubicle in the rear—an incubator. A tube of oxygen stood in a special rack.

For two weeks Baby R. lay in a water-jacketed metal tank,

held at an even temperature of 94 degrees. A slight pressure inside the tank helped him to breathe triple-filtered air, enriched with an extra supply of oxygen. At two-hour intervals a skillful nurse fed him mother's milk by nasal spoon. Food was passed through his nose because he was far too weak to spend energy swallowing a minute rubber tube which would have carried milk directly to his stomach. Not for weeks would he be strong enough to take a bottle.

After a fortnight in this darkened tank, Baby R. moved to a gas-heated incubator, furnished with glass sides. Gradually his appetite increased. Each day he could drink more of the mother's milk collected by a welfare agency and purchased by Dr. Couney, or of the milk supplied by one of the wet nurses who lived at the hospital. After a month in this incubator he graduated to the nursery. Two weeks here and he was ready to go home. He weighed seven pounds when his mother carried him away from the hospital. To almost any eyes this would represent a medical triumph. But to the mild, white-haired doctor who runs the place, it was a story he had seen thousands of times before.

Dr. Couney was born in Mülhausen, Germany, studied in Berlin and Leipzig, and did graduate work in Paris under Pierre-Constant Budin, great French gynecologist. Budin had pioneered in the field of raising incubator babies and wanted someone to demonstrate at the Berlin Exposition of 1896. He selected Couney for the job. The demonstration was a tremendous hit and Dr. Couney put on similar shows in London, Paris, and at the Trans-Mississippi Exposition in Omaha, in 1898. A few years later he settled permanently in this country, opening concessions on the Atlantic City Boardwalk, and at Coney Island.

Nearly all the 50 babies exhibited at the Fair last year came from New York hospitals. Of this group seven weighed less than two pounds, and 27 weighed between two and three pounds. There were three six-month babies, seven six-and-a-half-month babies. Out of the whole group of 50, 90 per cent survived. If allowances are made for three infants that died within 24 hours of admission the survival rate becomes 96 per cent!

In the early days distraught fathers brought him babies in shoe boxes, baskets, and even fish boilers. While he was exhibiting at Buffalo's Pan-American Exposition in 1901 a train conductor appeared one day. From Findlay, Ohio, he had brought a premature infant in a fruit basket, keeping it warm with pop bottles filled with hot water. Another time an undertaker delivered a baby given him as dead.

Perhaps the most dramatic moment in Dr. Couney's career came on January 29, 1907. His wife, six months pregnant, slipped and fell part way down a flight of stairs. Within a few hours she delivered a 2 ½-pound baby, whose chance for life appeared remote indeed. A blizzard was raging but Dr. Couney managed to hire a car for $50 and drive to his Coney Island establishment, closed for the winter. He got an incubator and arranged for mother's milk to be delivered by messenger at two-hour intervals. Daughter Hildegard survived.

Dr. Couney has not grown rich from his exhibits because of the staggering expense they involve. His hospital at the Fair cost $100,000. Incubators cost $700. Each baby requires about $5 worth of oxygen per day; and must have especially delicate garments made by French nuns. Coarse seams or heavy threads would cut their delicate bodies. The supply of mother's milk cost $1,300. Thirty-three adults were needed to care for 20 infants.

People who visit Couney's establishments are often skeptical. They repeatedly ask if the babies are alive. Children often ask if the babies are for sale. One man got his moral cockles up when he noted that a girl and boy baby were sleeping placidly together in the same incubator. But Dr. Couney's favorite visitor was an extremely puzzled young woman. She wanted to know how one should go about having a baby by incubation.

Dr. Couney's infants are, of course, the dramatic cases: the oddities. They are the ones almost sure to die if it weren't for his gentle ministrations. What of the other two and a quarter million children born each year in the United States? They, too, are getting an enormous amount of research attention. Medical men are trying to lessen the wrath of the diseases that strike them, psychologists are attempting to understand the subtle, life-shaping forces at work upon them, and nutritionists are seeking to determine what foods they should have.

Let us see what kind of a dollars-and-cents case can be made for this activity. Let us forget questions of mother love, questions of posterity. For the average family in moderate circumstances children represent the single largest capital investment.

The first cost is the cost of being born: the entrance fee into the world. This charge against the future citizen can vary through an extravagant range. If a woman requires the ministrations of a fashionable obstetrician she may pay $5,000 for his services. Her suite of rooms at the hospital will represent $2,000. Other expenses bring baby's cost up to $10,000 or more by the time he is moved into his elegant nursery. At the other end of the economic ladder a baby's initial cost may represent no cash outlay whatsoever.

Most American families lie between these extremes. A recent survey of the American Medical Association, covering 46 states, indicated that the median charge for a normal delivery is $45 to $100. Add other necessary costs to this fee and it develops that a baby costs the moderately well-to-do family in the neighborhood of $250. This is the first cost; the down payment, if you will. The real expenses begin once mother and infant arrive home from the hospital.

In their excellent study, *The Money Value of a Man,* Drs. Louis I. Dublin and Alfred J. Lotka, of the Metropolitan

Life Insurance Company, tabulated costs of raising a child to his eighteenth year. For the subject of their study they chose the family with yearly income of $2,500.

Each item of expense—health, clothing, recreation, etc.—was studied from masses of statistical data. Estimates were kept at the minimum. Education, from first grade to graduation from high school was allotted only $50. This sum covered cost of books. No charge was made for actual cost of the public schooling, borne by tax funds to which the family naturally had to contribute. Only $130 was allowed for recreation, this sum including movies, sports and vacations.

As they occur, these items are relatively insignificant. Yet they mount steadily to become respectable sums. By the time baby is one year old he represents an investment of $607. As he finishes the eighth grade the sum has risen to $7,200 and on graduation from high school stands at $10,485—which includes interest on expenditures at the rate of 3 $\frac{1}{2}$ per cent.

The largest items are represented by food at $2,755 and clothing and shelter at $3,333. Many other costs could be legitimately added to the total figure—cost of mother's time, for example. If she were allotted 25 cents an hour for three hours a day devoted to the care of a child, this would add about $5,000 to the cost of an 18-year-old. If the youngster postpones entering the gainful world to go to college the family outlay mounts still further, perhaps another $2,000. Regarded purely on a cost basis, child-bearing is America's largest industry. When we think in terms of the billions of dollars represented, research appropriations shrivel into insignificance.

We haven't space here for a complete survey of the work being done in this field. That would require many volumes. So we shall have to content ourselves with touching only a few of the high spots.

——— ——— ———

In New Haven, Connecticut, there is a trim, five-story Georgian building devoted solely to study of infants and small children. There are toys by the crate and furniture built to tot dimensions: gay red blocks and peg boards for infants, and fire engines for 3-year-olds. There are kitchens to prepare tasty dishes for the young and nurses who have words in their vocabularies besides "don't."

One room contains miniature pianos, a stage and a small open-air garden. Another pair of rooms, separated by a partition, contain identical furniture and identical toys for the entertainment of identical twins. Yet another contains a great gauze igloo in which there is a crib equipped with a toy tray.

Except for one peculiarity the building might be mistaken for a superbly equipped nursery. The peculiarity is this: wherever baby is and whatever he is doing, there is a pair of unseen eyes watching him through a one-way screen. Possibly a silent motion-picture camera is also making a record. This is the Yale Clinic of Child Development, which is conducting a magnificent study of the infant mind. The whole project started when a young psychologist decided to find out what went on inside baby's mind. It was like this:

Until a very few years ago people were apt to regard a baby as a living organism with certain animal appetites. He liked to eat, drink and sleep; laugh occasionally and cry frequently. But his mind appeared as a mass of disorganized, unpredictable cells.

Psychologists had studied the mind of the school-age child and of the adult. But the infant had received almost no attention. It was thus in 1911, when Dr. Arnold Gesell, then 31, came to Yale from California. He had barely had a chance to meet faculty members when he told his superiors he would like to conduct a study of the mind of the abnormal infant. They agreed.

Dr. Gesell had scarcely started his researches when one fact began to confront him wherever he turned. No one knew what a *normal* infant was! So how could you tell what an *abnormal* one was? The young psychologist set out to find the answer.

The first job was to find babies to study. The vital statistics bureau helped with this by furnishing the names of couples with infants. The next big job—and here human ingenuity was taxed to the utmost—was to find tests infants would respond to, as children and adults respond to I.Q. tests. At the beginning, there were no tracks to follow, so a method of trial and error was adopted.

Dr. Gesell began calling on new mothers. Patiently he would explain what he was trying to do. Would the mother help? Nearly always they agreed to cooperate.

Propping the babies up, Dr. Gesell would begin by placing before them simple objects: blocks, cups, spoons and rings. In a notebook he recorded the babies' reactions.

Finally he was working with scores of infants, making a monthly call on each one and noting its reactions to the simple toys he carried with him. Out of this arduous effort a pattern began to emerge. It developed that nearly all *normal* babies reacted alike to the several tests. Take the three red blocks, for example. At four weeks a baby would not notice them. At twelve weeks he would regard them briefly. At sixteen weeks he would stare at them for long periods. At twenty weeks the baby would try to pull them toward him, and at twenty-four would pick them up. At twenty-eight weeks the babies reached a peak of achievement: they would bang the blocks on the table and transfer them from hand to hand.

The most astonishing part of the work was that nearly every baby responded in precisely the same way and at precisely the same age. This indicated an exciting new fact: that the mind did develop at even stages and that simple tests could be used to determine normal progress. It also meant that for the first time a scientific explorer had made a start toward a better understanding of the infant mind.

Still Dr. Gesell wasn't satisfied. As he knew only too well, the human eye was fallible. There were, doubtless, many significant points he failed to note. So he began using motion-picture cameras to record reactions.

Let's see how all this works today. For sake of example let us suppose that you are about to adopt a baby—an adventure which involves an enormous risk. The fear that the infant may be of inferior intelligence haunts you. So before signing final papers you take the baby to the Yale Clinic.

Possibly it will be placed in a gauze igloo for observation. While silent observers watch, a nurse will put toys before the infant. One of these is the pill-in-the-bottle test. At one age the infant will regard the sugar pill intently, at another he will shake the bottle. At forty-four weeks he should be able to tip the bottle and get the pill out.

Possibly the crayon test will come next. The testing tools here are a crayon and a sheet of paper. At thirty-six weeks the infant should put the crayon in its mouth, at forty-four tap the paper with it and at fifty-two make scrawls.

The advantage of these tests is apparent: they detect any deviation in an infant from well established norms while the mind is still plastic enough to respond to simple psychiatric treatment. Furthermore, they are furnishing psychiatry with revealing new material. To illustrate, let us look at the case of a 14-year-old boy retarded mentally by a birth injury. A motion-picture camera study of this boy showed movement and characteristic position of his arms to be precisely those of a four-week-old infant. Presumably the boy's mental development had stopped at that point.

In many cases workers in the Yale Clinic can give a baby a clean bill of mental health immediately. Other times much longer observation is required. There are, it should be noted, no hard and fast rules. Dr. Gesell's tests merely act as guiding lines.

"Though it is impossible to cast a horoscope," Dr. Gesell says, "it is unnecessary to proceed blindly . . ."

The man who created this new branch of science is tall, pleasant and singularly handsome. A mop of white hair sets off a youthful face. About 1,000 infants and young children pass through his office each year before going on to the clinic.

Ofttimes Dr. Gesell can put his finger on the trouble with a difficult two-year-old immediately. Too many times the mother herself is at fault. Once she has mended her ways, baby's troubles cease. In more difficult cases, dozens of weekly observation periods are needed.

Yet another piece of recently completed work will illustrate the type of work being done by child psychologists. A widespread and foolish belief holds that childhood is a period without care or worry. Psychologists fail to concur. Children, they find, carry a burden of worry fully as great as that borne by adults. A poor report card is as upsetting as a business reverse and thoughts of growing up can be as painfully engrossing as a chronic illness. Children are more concerned about losing personal possessions than they are about the world coming to an end; and fret more about scoldings than they do about clothes. The possibility of death taking some member of the family is not nearly so troubling as the ever lurking threat of a spanking.

These are some of the findings of Drs. Rudolf Pintner, professor at Columbia University, and Joseph Lev, a WPA research worker. As originally planned, their project was designed to determine the amount of time children devote to worry. To get more practical results it was switched to investigate causes.

First step for the psychologists and their helpers was to get lists of random worries from a large group of children. To these the investigators added suggestions of their own. Result from a tabulation of 53 topics ranging from lateness for meals to death. This was then submitted to a group of 540 fifth and sixth graders in New York public schools. Half were boys, half girls.

The chief worry of the 12-year-old, it developed, was failing a test. Worry No. 2 was mother working too hard. (There was considerably less concern about father.) Third greatest worry was the possibility of mother getting sick. After this, worries of boys and girls diverged to meet again at the item causing least anguish of all: witches.

Boys were more uneasy about the house burning down than they were about kidnappers; and girls fretted far more about losing their fountain pens than about father decamping. Both groups were more concerned about being late for supper than they were about the world coming to an end; more worried by bad report cards than causing sadness to parents.

Two favorite subjects of maternal prodding—manners and talking too much—apparently represent so much wasted breath. Sleeplessness, robbers and lost friends caused more vexation than either of these topics.

By and large, girls were more self-sufficient than boys. They worried less about scoldings, ridicule and unfair treatment; but more about mother getting sick and lack of nice clothes.

One point was emphasized by the survey: the child is not the complete egoist that he is usually pictured to be. Groupings of chief worries indicated a marked feeling of responsibility for others. The family is the greatest cause of concern. School comes next and personal problems third.

A few figures indicate the relative positions of a few random worries:

Boys:

1. Failing a test
4. Being blamed for something you didn't do
8. Spoiling good clothes
16. Parents punishing you
24. Father losing his job
32. Bad marks in conduct
39. Death in the family
40. Making parents sad
46. Not having nice clothes
53. Witches

Girls:

2. Mother overworking
4. Being late for school
5. Getting sick
9. Father getting sick
14. Fighting with brother
16. Spoiling good clothes
18. Father losing his job
31. Death in the family
51. Not having pretty home
52. Getting married

"The excessive worry," conclusion of the investigators, "about school items would seem to indicate that our school system lays too much emphasis on *failing a test, having a poor report card, being late for school.* We cannot easily reduce children's worries about family matters, but we might very well do so in respect to school matters that are not very significant for the child's future growth and development."

CHAPTER XIII

IOWA PIONEERS

THE Iowa legislature voted down a bill to appropriate $25,000 for the study of children. The same afternoon it passed a bill carrying $25,000 to build a new sheep barn for the state fair grounds. The barn would be used one week a year.

Cora Bussey Hillis wept.

For fourteen years she had campaigned through the state. She drummed relentlessly on one theme: there were accepted standards by which one could judge cows, chickens, hogs. There were none for children. So far as exact scientific knowledge was concerned, the child was a complete unknown. Research alone could answer the questions that beset every mother.

Mrs. Hillis, wife of the mayor of Des Moines, logically approached the president of the state agricultural college. Couldn't he allot funds to study children, as he did to study farm animals? He was indignant. She marched to the president of the state university. He turned her out, saying he was more interested in a set of campanile chimes than in child research. She approached legislators. One sent her on her way with the statement that mother love was all a child needed. Angered, Mrs. Hillis replied that mother love wouldn't prevent a baby from dying of summer fevers, or prevent feeble-mindedness. The statesman wasn't interested.

A second refused his support on the ground that the child's place was in the home, not the laboratory; and a third made a dreary point. Scores of books had been written about children, he said, and no one had time to read them. Why collect information for others? The same logic could have been applied to medical research—and would have forestalled discovery of insulin, the liver treatment for pernicious anemia, and sulfanilamide. These arguments, you see, were made in the year 1915.

To say that Cora Hillis was not discouraged would be untrue. She was wretchedly, miserably discouraged. At the same time, she had "an overwhelming realization of the tremendous fact that every child born in the world is made or marred by the sort of care that it receives in its early life." Her driving desire was to find what this care consisted of; to secure solid, scientific facts such as were available on corn culture and sheep breeding.

Victory in her valiant fight came during the 1917 session of the legislature. War came to the aid of Mrs. Hillis. Throughout her campaign people had assured her that Iowa boys, raised in the sun and fed a nourishing diet were thoroughly sound and healthy. When Army doctors began to examine volunteers and draftees this thesis found no support. They found thousands of rejects in this supposedly healthy stock. Mrs. Hillis seized on this fact. Wasn't there room for more knowledge?

The legislature reluctantly agreed; passed her cherished bill. It voted funds to create the Iowa Child Welfare Research Station. Since then the station has achieved a worldwide reputation. It has pioneered in studies of nutrition, psychology and education. It developed the growth tables which today hang in every doctor's office, and did a thousand other jobs.

This bit of history is recapitulated for a single reason: most of our states today face the problem that confronted Iowa 24 years ago. There is a growing realization that a continuing democracy must inevitably rest on the unsteady shoulders of infants and small children. If this is true, then everything possible should be known about those who bear this responsibility. Are our children healthy, and do they have solid bones, good teeth? Are they intelligent and can they be made more intelligent? Do they receive proper schooling? In sum, what indeed are our children, and what has made them what they are?

Let's see how the Iowa station—first of its kind in the world—is getting answers to such questions. It is an object lesson in what other states might do if they had someone like the late Cora Hillis to prod reluctant legislatures to action.

The physical properties of the station aren't particularly prepossessing. There are a few scattered offices and laboratories in old East Hall, one of the buildings on the state university campus. And there are four nursery school cottages, all in need of paint, clustered in a group on East Market Street. The reputation of the station doesn't rest on this nondescript real estate; but on a realization in the minds of the 50 men and women who work there. To them the child is the least known and most exciting of all research subjects.

Problem No. 1, blocked out by Dr. Bird T. Baldwin, first station director, was to discover *how* infants and young children grew. At a casual glance it appears that such a question could be answered with a yardstick and a few children of assorted ages. But an astonishing number of complicating wrinkles appeared. Boys reached a temporary growth plateau at puberty; girls didn't. Added weight in an infant was represented largely by brain tissue and viscera. The same growth increment in a youth was largely bone and muscle, and in an adult, fat. Tens of thousands of measurements and years of patient effort went into the Baldwin-Wood growth tables now available for schools, clinics, doctors' offices.

Most emphasis in the station's work is placed on defining the normal child; what he is physically and intellectually. Second part is to find what forces produce superior children, and what forces produce inferior children.

The station has laboratories in the University Hospital's

obstetrical ward for studying infants from the moment of birth. (It even has equipment for phonetic analysis of the birth cry!) It has nursery, elementary and high schools for its own work.

State institutions for orphans, wayward and feeble-minded children all supply raw material for study. Work falls primarily into three categories: research; teaching; dissemination of new-found facts. The research program is the most important and interesting. See one of these projects.

When he accepted a position as psychologist on the station staff a few years ago Dr. Harold M. Skeels, small, dark, intense, was shocked to find the casualness with which children were adopted. The accepted practice elsewhere was to investigate mental and social background of true parents; then try to duplicate these conditions in foster homes. Such practice, it was felt, would prevent mentally inferior children from becoming unhappy burdens in superior homes. In Iowa such precautions were lacking. Children up for adoption were selected as casually as vegetables: because of attractive eyes, hair, or because of a nice smile.

Sure that he would find heartbreak, Skeels began checking children adopted under 6 months of age. He ran down case histories of 306 of these infants, most of whom were illegitimate. He and his helpers interviewed true mothers; and true fathers. Findings filled him with foreboding. Some of the mothers were feeble-minded, and some of the fathers were criminals. The true mothers had an average I.Q. of 85 (normal: 100), and the fathers, mostly unskilled laborers, were similarly backward. If old rules held children of such matings would be definitely inferior.

Then Skeels began invading foster homes, examining the adopted infants. For the better part the foster homes were of a superior sort. In many cases either husband or wife—or both—were college graduates. They had satisfied a deep yearning for children by adoption; and had expressed themselves in terms of love, care and attention of an order generally higher than that encountered with most true parents. Response of the children to such treatment? In one group of 2-year-olds Skeels discovered an average I.Q. of 116! A group of 6-year-olds averaged 111!

Intelligence, it appeared, wasn't fixed irrevocably at birth. An earlier study in the Kentucky mountains showed that normally intelligent infants could be dragged downward to low intellectual levels by their drab surroundings. This study indicated that the process could be reversed.

Further proof was developed by Dr. George D. Stoddard, director of the station and head of Iowa's graduate college. Stoddard, 44, is big, baldish and pleasantly informal. No ivory tower theoretician, he speaks clearly and makes his points in language easily understood outside narrow academic precincts.

He has a burning conviction that intelligent care can produce superior human beings and is devoting his energy to defining the care required. But Stoddard himself is the best expression of his beliefs.

"Children," he says, "do not just grow up. They are cultivated. The child is an intricate mechanism which doesn't stay put. He keeps changing into something else. The child himself is the story of his life, and he has not had too much to do with its writing. Almost everything the child does or thinks is a response to something, to somebody. If we wholly like the emerging result, we say 'well done.' But if we reject or abhor the misshapen, misguided outcome as a drunk, tramp, or criminal, we wash our hands and squeal of the wickedness of God's plan.

"These outcomes are the extremes. Most of the time the child moves to some dead center of ability and adjustment. He grows up so-so, learns so-so, and carries out his life so-so. This is the slow, deep-lying tragedy which marks the distinction between what the human race is, and what it might be.

It is a resultant, not so much from defective genes, as from spiritless education and bleak social opportunity."

One study sponsored by Stoddard illustrates his point and supports the Skeels work. Stoddard is impatient with people who arbitrarily select the age of six as the point at which a child's education should begin. Why not, he asks, say schooling should begin at eight or fifteen? Since the Iowa work is based on research and not idle theorizing, Stoddard set out to find whether or not he was right in this belief.

As locale for his study he selected the Iowa Soldiers' Orphans' Home at Davenport. Due to press of circumstances at the Davenport orphanage, children under six got little attention. They existed in a dull, stultifying atmosphere awaiting the time they could begin school. They had few toys to play with, and no activity to teach self-reliance. Their coats were hung on hooks too high for them to reach; and attendants aided them in making their toilet with fixtures meant for adults.

The youngsters had no pride in possessions. Clothes worn one week might be given to another child when they came back from the laundry the following week. There were few toys.

From the 700 children in the orphanage, Stoddard and his helpers selected two groups as nearly identical as possible. The controls would remain in the orphanage routine; the others would attend nursery school.

At the nursery school, a pleasant home-like structure set apart from the institution's cottages, everything was built to fit the child. Youngsters fortunate enough to attend saw the world as a new and exciting place. They had paints, toys and clay. They listened to stories and took walks through the woods, examining bugs, leaves, and flowers.

Response to their new environment was indicated at the termination of the project. The pre-school group had gained nearly five points in the I.Q.'s; the controls had lost an almost exactly similar number. Three children from the control group eventually wound up in a home for the feeble-minded; none in the pre-school group did. Here was the strong support Stoddard needed for his beliefs. Note in passing that as a result of this work the orphanage adopted a pre-school program for *all* children.

Another project has glowing possibilities. In effect it is a scientifically exact appraisal of all school children in five Iowa counties: one county in the center of the state and one in each of the four corners. Each of 28,000 children has been checked for mal-occlusions of teeth and their relation to speech defects; intelligence, aptitude, general health and vigor.

Portable recording machines make records of speech defects for analysis, and an ingenious device checks hearing. Forty children at a time sit with earphones clamped to their heads and write down the words and numbers that come to them. The voice grows fainter and they can no longer hear. The point at which sound fades to nothing is a measure of their hearing ability. Such tests ofttimes explain why the little boy placed in the back row appears to be dull. When moved to the front row he may become an honor student.

Working with a limited budget, Stoddard knew it was hopeless to try and correct the disorders discovered in 9,000 of the 28,000 children thus examined. But whenever a child was found needing glasses, dental attention, or surgery, word was passed to the school superintendent who in turn passed it along to parents or some philanthropic organization. Hence the project was largely one of discovery. But it also has a larger purpose. If authorities in each of the state's 99 counties can be impressed with the rather shocking fact that *nearly a third of all children need some remedial attention,* perhaps they can be persuaded to take action. Stoddard would like them all to undertake surveys similar to the one conducted in the five counties; and then take necessary steps to correct ailments discovered.

Still another project attempted to answer some of the puzzling questions presented by fascism. It was conducted by Dr. Kurt Lewin, a refugee from Germany and a veteran of four years' World War service with the German army.

Dr. Lewin set up his problem. Why not create conditions of authority which would approximate fascism, democracy and anarchy? Then subject the psychologist's best guinea pig— the child—to those conditions and see how he reacted? If experiments sound unnecessarily cruel to the children involved, the reader should be patient for a moment or so.

Lewin, with the help of Ronald Lippitt and Ralph White, selected children from Iowa City grade schools. The children were told that clubs were being formed where they would make model airplanes, theatrical masks, furniture. Those who wanted to join should raise their hands. From those who volunteered, four groups of five children were selected. Scholastic ability, social relationships, family background and other such factors were checked for each child in an effort to make groups as nearly alike as possible.

It was up to leaders—graduate students in psychology—to duplicate three sets of conditions. At six club meetings the ten-year-olds would work under democratic conditions. In a second period they would be under authoritarian or fascist conditions; and for the balance of the time under laissez faire or anarchy. Ten observers kept club meetings under minute observation. Stenographic records were made of all conversation, and the movie camera made another record.

Under authoritarian conditions the leader determined all policy and directed all actions, whereas in democracy the leader gave club members various alternatives and let them vote on procedure. Under anarchy the leader answered only those questions that were put directly to him.

During the fascist club periods the children seldom smiled and rarely spoke. The same air of tenseness prevailed that many tourists have noted in Germany. Children did what they were told to do but stopped work immediately the leader left the room. Under democracy they were talkative and friendly. The presence of the leader made little difference to them. They continued work whether he was in the room or not. Children discussed problems and assumed the jobs for which they were best fitted. Under anarchy there was a lot of horse play but little work. This spirit of robust freedom in the anarchist groups, gradually gave way to complete boredom.

Statistical summations gave a revealing picture. There were 40 times as many hostile acts under fascist conditions as under democracy. Under fascism 70 per cent of all utterances were "I" centered, rather than "we" centered. For the democratic groups this figure was only 30 per cent. Under fascism there was marked submission to the leader and "scapegoat" situations arose frequently. At different times, the whole group ganged up on a single luckless youngster making life so unpleasant that he dropped club membership. Work accomplished, negligible under anarchy, was about the same for both fascism and democracy. This fact surprised sponsors of the experiment. They expected authoritarian efficiency to far outstrip democracy.

Votes and interviews after the last club meetings gave more facts. Children invariably elected their democratic leaders most popular, although that same leader might have performed the authoritarian rôle with another club. Only one out of 20 children—the son of an army officer—preferred fascism to democracy. Seven out of ten preferred anarchy to fascism. A typical comment on an authoritarian leader: "We didn't have any fun with him." Of an anarchist leader: "He was too easygoing."

Disposal of the products made offered another sidelight. In an orderly manner the democratic groups voted to give the leader one of the theatrical masks the club had made, and voted disposition of the others. In authoritarian groups there was much bickering. One child finally snatched a mask and, in a fury, smashed it to pieces.

The reader may draw whatever parallels he will between facts turned up by these experiments and conditions as they exist in totalitarian countries. For his part, Dr. Lewin is cautious, but one thing seems to be clear. Best results in the field of education will come, not from the iron-fisted schoolmaster of tradition, and not from radical progressive schools which allow complete child freedom. The experiments indicate that a moderate compromise will best serve to cultivate individual initiative.

Information gathered by the Iowa station would be of little value if it were made the exclusive property of dieticians, child psychologists and other professional people. Because of this the station spends a large part of its budget in getting findings into the home. It has distributed over 700,000 popular pamphlets and bulletins. It conducts child study classes over the state which thus far have enrolled 20,000 mothers, and sends out a syndicated column printed in 160 newspapers. Its radio programs go out twice weekly and 60 Iowa towns have organized listening groups which follow the radio program with discussion. Typical programs: Anger and Jealousy; Health Hazards of Childhood; Sex Education. The same program is broadcast in other states; and even in Ceylon where it is sponsored by a former station student.

As a matter of course Iowa people call the station whenever a problem with their children arises. A mother notes a tendency to stutter in her small son. The station supplies exact information on what she should do, and suggests that she bring the child in if improvement isn't noted. Another woman has a behavior problem with her 9-year-old daughter; and a third wishes to know what consequences are to be expected from a marriage of first cousins. An anxious father wants to know how to break his infant son of thumb-sucking;

and a hopeful but old-fashioned school principal is desirous of knowing the latest methods of punishment. Such are the questions asked by the thousands of people who write and call the station for trustworthy advice about problems presented by their children.

Dictator countries are interested in *quantity* of children produced—children are the raw material for conquest. Democracies should be interested in *quality*. Iowa has pointed the way. Cost of the work has been meagre in light of achievements. Since the start the station has stood the state only a little over $600,000. Outside philanthropies have added about a million more. Currently, the work is costing about $70,000 a year. This is surely a small sum to pay for a better understanding of children. The cost trails into insignificance when one remembers the larger purpose of the work: to right "the tragedy . . . of what the human race is, and what it might be."

CHAPTER XIV

SANITARY DIMPLE

BECAUSE of carelessness, poverty or ignorance, tens of thousands of people die needlessly each year. Unprotected infants are strangled by diphtheria. Syphilis and pneumonia destroy adults. Cancer takes an unnecessary toll among older people. This is little better than mass murder. Yet . . . who is to blame? Unfortunately, pure carelessness in a great many cases. No better case can be cited than that of smallpox.

There is a general disposition to think of smallpox as a horrible specter of the Middle Ages; a disease which has graciously vanished from the earth. Mark that down as false. This year there will be something like a quarter of a million cases of smallpox in the world. Enough will die to populate a city the size of Lexington, Kentucky.

A chart which hangs in Washington indicates that our own enlightened country may be ripe for a grisly harvest. For five years now smallpox has been on a steady upward march and this year thousands of people will go to bed with the disease which should by now be completely eradicated.

These figures are appalling. There is no reason—get that straight, *no* reason—for existence of this disease. Against the cruel, disfiguring, and often lethal wrath of smallpox, science has provided the most perfect protection that it has brewed for any disease. Light has been available since that day in 1798 when a crossroads pill roller, Dr. Edward Jenner of Berkeley, England, dug into his own pocket to pay for printing a tract which medical journals had rejected. The story that tract told was brilliant in its simplicity: if men would squeeze a little juice from a pock on a sick cow, and scratch a little of that juice into their arms, it wouldn't be necessary for them to die of the disease which regularly sent one out of every ten people born to the grave.

In the past 143 years millions of people have heeded Jenner's message and have been protected. Others, through carelessness, ignorance or superstition, haven't. In India the disease takes a frightful annual toll because natives believe smallpox of divine origin and refuse vaccination. African blacks escape vaccination because of ignorance. With Americans carelessness is the villain.

It isn't likely that more than a few dozen U.S. citizens will die this year of smallpox. But should all those people die in a railroad wreck caused by utter carelessness, the hue and cry would be deafening. There is absolutely no consolation in the fact that deaths are at present small in number. This is a reflection on the potency of the strain of smallpox now at large, rather than on a credit to the good care people take of their bodies.

In epidemics of variola major—that's the medical name for the severe type—as many as seven out of every ten stricken will perish. Then why, you may ask, bother about this new smallpox if it isn't the killer type? On the surface it looks like a feeble public enemy indeed if it can't take as many lives as firecrackers or infected stubbed toes. Look under the surface and you'll see the point.

The significant thing about the present mild smallpox is that it indicates the immunity level of the population is low. If it can spread with the ease that it does, variola major would go like wildfire. Therefore, the recent rise in the number of cases should be regarded as a possible harbinger of calamitous things to come, rather than as a particularly serious problem within itself.

It is false solace to suppose that vaccination is responsible for lessening the virulence of the smallpox microbe. Mild epidemics have been noted scores of times before. As early as

1782 Jenner reported on an epidemic of non-fatal smallpox in Gloucestshire. Then the severe type returned to kill 2,000,000 people in Russia in a single year. On the other hand, there is no reason to believe the present mild strain will develop into a major strain. The wild, crazy type of smallpox, always present somewhere in the world, will be introduced from the outside.

Classical smallpox is a disease horrible to behold. Let's forget squeamishness for a moment and take a good look at it; get a fixed picture of this enemy of mankind. It is caused by a virus. How this potent dynamite gets about, no one is quite sure. Apparently it can travel for at least a few feet through the air. It is present in the body discharges of the sick. It must be able to get about in a hundred ways. Otherwise there is no explaining the cases that appear spontaneously, without the stricken person having had any intimate contact with another sick person.

Once this stuff is in an unprotected—unvaccinated—body, it grows and multiplies for as little as eight and as many as 21 days before anything happens. The infected person is unaware of the violence brewing in his body. Then one day he has a headache. And a backache. Body temperature shoots up to 104 or 105 degrees F. In this stage no doctor can be sure what is the matter. It might be nothing more than a bad cold. Then clinching evidence appears—papules.

These little red welts crop up along the hairline, and on the feet and hands. Smallpox is a "centrifugal" disease—whirl a man by his umbilicus and the first lesions appear where the centrifugal pull is greatest. In the following few days these papules spread over the body.

In the next stage the papules fill with water, become vesicles. Features are so distorted that the face is almost unrecognizable. Gradually these water blisters fill with pus. Then crusts form which may take as long as 40 days to drop off—drop off, leaving a pitted skin and possibly impaired vision or even blindness.

This is the disaster millions of people are courting by not availing themselves of good Dr. Jenner's protection. And no other protection exists. No amount of cleanliness or good living helps in the slightest degree. What is this magic brew?

It is made by shaving a patch of belly hair off a calf, and directly inoculating the calf with the virus of smallpox. The exudate from the sores that results is collected, purified, mixed with glycerine and packed in ampoules. A new procedure, developed at the Rockefeller Institute, eliminates the calf. Virus for vaccine is grown in a test tube, the disease organisms getting nourishment from the embryos of unhatched chicks. It is also grown in fertile eggs.

A tiny amount of the material from either of these sources will, when pressed into the skin, set up a mild infection. This stimulates the body to build antibodies. The vaccination mark is nothing more than a deliberately created pock, a sanitary dimple.

Although basic principles haven't changed since Jenner's time, methods of vaccination have. Doctors no longer "scarify"—break—the skin. Instead, they place a drop of vaccine no larger than an eighth of an inch in diameter on the arm. A needle, held crosswise to the arm, is jiggled up and down about 30 times, the point merely depressing the skin. Resultant tension pulls some of the vaccine into the arm. The whole process requires no more than a few seconds and at no time is blood drawn. The vaccination scar resulting is no larger than a shoe button—a happy contrast to the whitish patch of skin as large as a nickel that resulted from vaccinations a decade or so ago.

When people object too strenuously to even this insignificant badge of protection, vaccinations can be made on the leg. The only possible drawback here is that, because of the more general presence of perspiration on the legs, better medical attention is required. There is also the remote possibility of contamination by street dust.

One cannot deny that there are occasional complications to vaccination. The most severe complication is tetanus—lockjaw—which is even more serious than smallpox itself. Fortunately, there will be hundreds of thousands of uneventful vaccinations for every case of tetanus. And even these scattered cases are wholly unnecessary.

Dr. Charles Armstrong, big, breezy veteran of a score of the United States Public Health Service's campaigns against disease, nailed this fact solidly down. It was as pretty a job of investigation as you would ever care to see. Armstrong laid his facts out on the table. The spores which cause tetanus are anaerobic, that is to say they thrive in the absence of air. They also like a warm, moist environment. And where did one find these conditions? Under those infernal bunion plasters that doctors insisted on plastering over vaccinations!

The case looked good on paper, but scientific journals have no interest whatsoever in paper cases. Armstrong set out to back up his thesis. All over the country he broadcast a message: would health officers let him know when a case of post-vaccination tetanus cropped up?

It took months to collect 123 cases of tetanus but results were lovely to behold. Fifty-eight of those cases developed where doctors had hermetically sealed the vaccination with "shields"—rings of cotton fiber; 46 had been covered with gauze; 17 with bunion pads and two with adhesive and gauze. There had not been a single case of tetanus where dressings had been omitted entirely!

Armstrong checked these findings with monkeys. First, he shaved patches of fur off the frisky little animals, vaccinated them and deliberately rubbed *clostridium tetani*—the tetanus microbe—into the wound. Not one case of tetanus resulted, as long as the festering vaccination mark was unbandaged.

Next, Armstrong had to find what would happen if the vaccinations were bandaged. That was a job. ("If you want to spend a painful afternoon, try and put a bandage on a monkey that he can't pull off.") Armstrong solved this one by pressing the smallpox vaccine—and the tetanus microbes—into the skin between the shoulder blades. Then he wrapped a tight, corset bandage around those firecracker packages of teeth and claws. Eight out of ten of the monks in this group got tetanus! Armstrong had proved that any case of post-vaccination tetanus could be charged to the carelessness of the operator.

If the negligible number of tetanus cases that appear today represented the only case against vaccination, the case would be scarcely worth consideration. Another—and a far more serious—case is presented by those misguided people—the anti-vaccinationists. By using a tool unavailable to the medical profession—the emotional appeal—they have been able to influence legislation and lead large segments of the population away from safety.

The appeal of these groups, runs to a pattern. Why, they ask, "contaminate" the blood with "pus." Vaccine, of course, isn't pus, and vaccination could hardly be considered as "contamination." Blatantly they charge that vaccination is a means of spreading syphilis, cancer and tuberculosis; neglecting, of course, to mention that calves which furnish vaccine are immune to syphilis, are rigidly and positively tested for tuberculosis and are utterly incapable of transmitting cancer. Yet, the pseudo-scientific revival meetings put on by the anti-vaccinationists are popular. They generally include a weeping mother who professes to have lost her baby by vaccination, another who has—mysteriously—had her child crippled, and a lawyer who, in his best murder trial voice, explains legal aspects of vaccination.

At these shows figures are juggled shamelessly. The fact is cited that there are several million vaccinations each year and that there are only a few thousand cases of smallpox. This is used to *prove* that vaccination is needless, instead of accepting it in a more logical light to indicate that vaccination is responsible for keeping the number of cases low. After making this glaringly inaccurate statement, a statement which gullible listeners rarely question, performers go on to charge vaccination with actually causing smallpox! They state that when there is a great deal of vaccination there is a great deal of smallpox. This is indubitably true. But the rise in the number of vaccinations is caused by people rushing for protection. To combat this appeal, doctors cannot weep and moan on the platform. But they can present a body of convincing statistics. Prior to the United States occupation of the Philippines there were 50,000 smallpox deaths a year. Annually a temporary smallpox hospital was thrown up in Manila; a hospital from which few emerged alive.

After an aggressive campaign of vaccinations, deaths dropped to nearly zero by 1909. Then the native legislature listened to the pleas of anti-vaccinationists, and allowed the campaign to come to a standstill. Smallpox came back with a terrible vengeance. In the epidemic of 1918–'19 there were 66,000 deaths. Ninety per cent of those deaths were in the non-immune population made up of children under ten years of age. After this dark visitation, vaccination was resumed and in 1925 there was only one recorded case of smallpox in the islands. That one was imported from China.

If a still more convincing argument is needed, one has only to consult the incidence rate of the disease in the United States as shown by a ten-year study. In the decade which included 1937 there were 35 cases per 100,000 population in states with no compulsory vaccination laws. In states which demanded vaccination of every school child there were 4.1 cases—only an eighth as much smallpox!

The late Sir William Osler, a great writer and a brilliant diagnostician made an offer which a thousand doctors would willingly duplicate:

"I will go into the next severe epidemic with ten selected

vaccinated persons and ten unvaccinated persons. I should prefer to choose the latter; three members of parliament, three anti-vaccination doctors if they could be found, and four anti-vaccination propagandists. And I will make the promise neither to jeer nor to jibe when they catch the disease, but to look after them as brothers, and for four or five who are certain to die I will try and arrange the funerals without the pomp and ceremony of an anti-vaccination demonstration."

Let no one enjoy the smug assurance that the great killer either can't or won't return. Variola major struck Colorado in 1922 and left 1,086 dead, and took a minor swipe at Detroit in 1925, killing 175. The Minnesota epidemic of the winter 1924–'25 took 505 lives. Thousands who had been exposed rushed for—and got—protection.

The vaccine mercifully produces protective factors at a more rapid speed than the disease itself can manufacture its killing juice. Hence, if one could always be sure of the time at which he was exposed to the disease, there would be little need for advance protection. But no one *can* be sure, and not more than one in a dozen people who get the disease have more than the vaguest notion as to where they contracted it.

Waiting for this calamity to strike before getting protection is foolhardy indeed. It is especially foolhardy in light of the fact that a shockingly large non-immune population exists. One spark—a spark in the form of an imported case of variola major—could set off the conflagration.

Infants should be vaccinated within a few weeks of birth. At this age reactions are slight. There is no chance of the baby scratching his vaccination and in turn scratching other skin openings such as insect bites—thereby setting up secondary vaccinations and making permanent scars in undesirable places. Furthermore, this procedure corrects the general, but foolish practice of allowing a child to go unvaccinated until he enters school, thereby passing the most susceptible years of his life without protection. People vaccinated as infants generally have no reaction whatsoever to subsequent vaccinations necessary every five to ten years.

Anyone in doubt as to his smallpox immunity can take a simple test which will give a positive answer. A doctor simply makes three minor pricks in the skin of the arm, about an inch apart. On the two outer ones he rubs the tiniest drops of vaccine. If the individual is protected the two pricks thus treated will take on the pinkish hue of a mosquito bite within 48 hours.

If there is no reaction, there is no protection. That individual needs vaccination; needs that glowing little badge of protection on the arm which indicates he has been wise enough to avail himself of the positive knowledge medicine has provided.

CHAPTER XV

COTTONFIELD CLINIC

CARELESSNESS accounts for a great deal of disease. We fail to avail ourselves of the protection the research man has labored to provide. Other times the rigid science of economics steps in. A figure or so will clarify this point. To feed a human being adequately for a year costs $150. Allowing for an average of five people to the family this makes a food bill of $750 per year. Yet 27 per cent of the population is below this income level. For them health is a purchasable commodity and they don't have the price.

Come along to the back country of the Deep South and see these people. And see what is being done for them by an isolated group. In making this trip it isn't the author's desire to suggest that the situation can be cured by private charitable agencies. The problem is far too big for such haphazard solution. Our sole purpose of observing this particular piece of work is to indicate *need*. Suggestion of a solution for the problem is outside the province of this book.

Witness a scene on a back road in the fabulous Mississippi Delta; a scene no casual traveler will ever witness. Several hundred Negroes are lounging about in the smothering July heat. All kinds of Negroes: babies in arms, old men twisted with rheumatism, expectant mothers, husky young field hands. As they loaf or munch sandwiches or drink warm soda pop, they watch what is happening under the cottonwood trees, where a dozen colored women in starched white uniforms are at work.

Here is a table covered with a white sheet—a table made by laying an unhinged door across a pair of sawhorses. On the table bubbles a sterilizer. A Negro nurse quickly, quietly, takes a hypodermic syringe from the sterilizer, draws it full of toxoid, and shoots it into the arm of a frightened five-year-old. That little Negro girl will never have diphtheria. At the other end of the table another Negro nurse is pressing vaccine into the arm of a howling baby. There's one victim less for smallpox.

Off in one corner of the cottonwood grove a Negro woman dentist is filling teeth. Power for her portable drill comes from a treadle. In another corner a Negro interviewer listens patiently while an old granny describes the misery of chills and fevers that racks her bones. No microscopic examination is needed here. Malaria. And quinine will stop it. Farther off a Negro woman doctor snaps a glass seal off the needle end of a Keidel tube. The tube's vacuum sucks up blood from the arm of a young fellow—blood which will be tested for the spirochetes of syphilis. The strapping young field hand is neither frightened nor ashamed that he may have this disease. "Bad blood," he calls it—or "old dog." Here in this lost province of cotton's kingdom, where one will find few either of the taboos or medical blessings of civilization, syphilis is hideously common, and carries no social stigma.

The spectacle of wretchedly ill, suffering, and ignorant Negroes is only too easy to find in our America. Denied education and kept at low economic levels, the Negro in the past has had to depend on the white man for whatever medical care he got. Pioneer work by the Rosenwald Fund has helped change this. Hospitals have opened to allow the Negro internships. Scores of rural counties have added Negro public health nurses, and large-scale training programs for midwives have been launched. The Negro's hunger for health—far more acute than found among whites at similar economic levels—is getting some satisfaction.

The cottonfield clinic is simply an isolated example of the Negro taking the initiative himself. It is sponsored by Alpha

Kappa Alpha, a sorority of Negro college women and is absolutely unique. Dr. Thomas Parran, surgeon-general of the United States Public Health Service, calls it one of the best jobs of volunteer public health work he has ever seen.

For six years now these women have volunteered each summer to take health to a place where it is desperately needed—rural Mississippi. They have given up their summer vacations; driven their own cars over bumpy roads to set up clinics wherever there was room—in schools, churches, out of doors. Annual budgets drawn from dues paid by the sorority's 2,200 Negro members and from the donations of its 125 chapters have yet to exceed $2,500. Personnel, largely composed of Negro professional women, shifts each year. Workers who come from all parts of the country donate their services. Tuskegee sent a Negro public health nurse. Boston sent a dentist and Washington a physician. A colored nursery-school teacher from Philadelphia helped with secretarial work and so did another teacher from Norfolk. Each of the twelve workers is allowed $10.50 a week for board, lodging, and laundry; and the sorority supplies gasoline for their cars. Otherwise every cent appropriated goes for medical supplies.

On time donated to help their own people, this remarkable group has immunized about 14,500 children against diphtheria and smallpox; treated thousands of adults for malaria, syphilis and other diseases; provided expectant mothers and rickety children with such protective food concentrates as dried milk, yeast, and vitamins.

The project began in 1933, when a member of the sorority, Ida L. Jackson, Negro junior high school teacher of Oakland, California, heard a group of singers from Saints Industrial School of Lexington, Mississippi. A speaker who accompanied the young girls described conditions among colored share-croppers in the cotton country. It was a story of poverty and ignorance, inevitable handmaidens of disease; a story of leaky-roofed shanties without screens or privies; and of family incomes of less than $50 a year.

Miss Jackson investigated. Everything was as it had been pictured. At the annual meeting of her sorority she made a novel proposal for philanthropy. Why not send a delegation of volunteer teachers to Lexington, Mississippi—home of the Saints School—to conduct extension courses for teachers, and classes for illiterate adults? Funds were forthcoming and six teachers went to Mississippi for six weeks in the summer of 1934. At the end of their work all agreed they were on the wrong track. The southern Negro was, first of all, in need of better health. Syphilis and tuberculosis given him by the white man were taking a frightening toll. Infant and maternal mortality were inordinately high, and the deficiency diseases that accompany bad diet were needlessly prevalent. Take care of these things first, the teachers suggested, and let education come later. The sorority appropriated $1,500 for medical work in 1935 and appointed Dr. Dorothy Boulding Ferebee, Negro general practitioner in Washington, to head a medical mission.

Dr. Ferebee, member of a family that has produced several generations of lawyers, was born in Norfolk, Virginia, and grew up in Boston. She attended Simmons College and took medicine at Tufts, graduating *cum laude*. From a large number of women who volunteered for service she selected a group of eleven. Plans were carefully drawn. The group would conduct one central clinic at Lexington during the inactive summer "lay-by"—between cotton chopping and picking. Work would be restricted to giving children under twelve protection against smallpox and diphtheria. Such a program would be least likely to arouse the southern planters' ever-present fear of "outside agitators."

When these women arrived in Holmes County a heartbreaking setback awaited them. Planters refused to allow Negroes to attend the clinics. Dr. Ferebee asked help of the county health officer. Would he drive with her to see the landowners? He readily agreed. For several days they went through the county. The story Dr. Ferebee told the planters was convincing. She was interested only in health. Wasn't it to the landowners' advantage to share this interest? Wasn't it better to have children protected against diphtheria than to have them die or aid in spreading the disease?

In only one case did these arguments fail. All the other planters agreed to allow the work to begin—on one condition. The group would have to conduct its clinics on plantations, under the owners' watchful eyes. The plan for central clinics which farm workers could reach by foot, mule or truck had to be abandoned.

This meant mobile clinics. It meant that the Negro health missionaries would have to make arrangements to refrigerate biological supplies, storing them in ice plants over the country and withdrawing them only as they were needed. And it meant that doctors and nurses trained in the use of adequate hospital facilities would have to learn to use whatever was at hand. It should be noted that in spite of added complications this turned out to be by far the better plan. The clinic reached people in isolated districts who could never have trekked miles to a central location.

After a few days spent making arrangements and drawing a schedule of stops, the work began. That summer the six-car caravan covered 5,300 miles in Holmes County. The women workers administered 2,000 doses of diphtheria toxoid and 3,000 doses of smallpox vaccine.

Fearing that the sorority might not have funds to finance the work indefinitely, Dr. Ferebee decided to leave Holmes County, and the second summer's work was done in nearby Bolivar County. She wanted to spread the effort of her group as far as possible in relieving the appalling conditions encountered.

Bolivar County is midway between Memphis and Vicksburg. Seventy-five per cent of the county's 80,000 population is Negro. It has a staggering health problem. Very likely the county's syphilis rate—30 per cent of the population—is exceeded nowhere else in the United States. In 1938, the 33 physicians in the county reported nearly 400 cases of pellagra. Hundreds went unreported. That same year nearly 1,000 cases of dysentery were recorded. The tuberculosis death rate among Negroes is three times as high as among whites. Conditions for tuberculosis are ideal; 10 per cent of the houses average three or more people per bed!

But these appalling figures must not be blamed on the laxity of Bolivar County's health department. It is one of the best and most active in the state—on an annual budget which allows 25 cents per citizen for health work. One dollar is considered barely adequate in other communities. At the head of the county's health department is Dr. R. D. Dedwylder, 58. He is a veteran of the Rockefeller Foundation's famous hookworm commission, and of the International Health Board's malaria project. He worked with Dr. Joseph Goldberger, a medical immortal, when that great genius was tracking down the cause of pellagra; he was the first doctor in the South to use toxin-antitoxin to ward off diphtheria.

When Dr. Dedwylder set up the county organization in 1920 it was usual for schools to close at least once a year because of diphtheria epidemics. A few years before this, a survey showed that over 80 per cent of the people had malaria parasites in their blood. Considering risks too great, insurance companies had taken the drastic step of refusing to write policies for anyone living in Bolivar County.

With evangelical zeal Dedwylder preached screening and drainage to cut the malaria toll. He is now in the midst of a syphilis campaign which is a model for the whole South. He and his small staff (ten people) are conducting ten free clinics a week, which treat from 600 to 2,000 people. School children are excused from classes to attend and field workers are brought in by truck. Last year Dr. Dedwylder personally gave

25,000 hip shots of bismuth, while his assistants gave several times as many arm shots of arsenicals. The pace which he set for himself is largely responsible for the halving of Bolivar's death rate in the past two decades.

Dedwylder, a white man born and raised amid all the racial prejudices of the Deep South, had no inhibitions about working with Negroes. He gave the Alpha Kappa Alpha group the cooperation that is absolutely essential to eventual solution of the Negro health problem. From Dedwylder's point of view their arrival was a boon. They could tell the story of health to their own people in a language which would be understood. Dedwylder drew up clinic schedules in advance of their arrival, printed posters and had them tacked in stores and on hundreds of fence posts.

Everything was ready for the women workers when they appeared. They set up headquarters in the all-Negro town of Mound Bayou. Word of the mission's arrival went out over the country; preachers spoke of it from the pulpit and plantation owners told their workers.

For the first year in Bolivar the chief job was immunizing children against smallpox and diphtheria. Although these treatments were compulsory for school children, only 65 per cent of the Negro children of school age were actually in school. Furthermore, cotton-belt Negroes migrate endlessly in search of better conditions. An annual labor turnover of 30 per cent made it imposible to catch all the youngsters in this transient population.

Year by year, as the proportion of the population protected has risen, emphasis on this part of the work has dwindled and the medical workers have shifted to other fields. Here is a sample day.

By seven in the morning clinic workers have fresh linen, medical supplies, and health literature stowed in the back seats of their cars and are ready to start. Since they work anywhere within a 45-mile radius of Mound Bayou it may take two hours to drive to the spot selected for the day's clinic. Many people will be waiting. Some have been there since dawn.

The clinical assistants begin interviewing. One by one Negroes march up to give histories. An old man thinks he was born in Alabama, but doesn't know when. A young woman enters her two divorces in the record; divorces achieved by a "script" painfully written out by a literate neighbor. Youngsters, saucer-eyed with fear, watch other terrified children submit to vaccination. Babies stop nursing long enough to howl defiance at the hot sun, then turn back to their mothers' breasts. This is the cottonfield clinic; vaguely a social engagement, but more particularly a gathering of poor people come to seek that elusive thing, good health, which they hope the "doctor women" will give them.

The large majority of these Negroes have never before in their lives had medical attention; and 25 per cent of them will die with no doctor to attend their final illnesses. They were brought into the world by midwives and from then on had to shift for themselves. As infants they had milk if their mothers could supply it. If not, they sucked rinds of "fat back" and drank water sweetened with molasses. Such a diet explains legs bowed by rickets.

Eighty per cent of the children have diseased tonsils and adenoids. The clinic workers can do nothing about this because they have no surgical facilities. And there is little chance that parents of the child can do anything either. The median cash income of the colored share-cropper is $38 a year. There are just two Negro doctors in the county and no hospital for the black man. There is a similarly hopeless outlook for adults with such chronic ailments as hernia, arthritis, rheumatism. But elsewhere the picture is not so dark.

Thanks to excellent cooperation from the county, treatment for syphilis is provided by the clinic. A blood sample drawn by one of the clinic nurses goes to the state laboratory at Jackson, which handles a quarter of a million blood samples every year. If the sample reacts positively to the Wassermann test, treatment is immediately begun. After clinic workers have finished their summer's work, treatment is continued by the county, perhaps for as long as 40 weeks. Likewise, quinine is passed out for the long courses of malaria treatments.

In pre-natal cases mothers are examined thoroughly. If unusual conditions are discovered word is passed along to one of the county's 130 Negro midwives. If the mother is syphilitic, treatment is rushed to prevent her passing the disease along to her baby. Dental care, of necessity, is limited. But each child gets a free toothbrush and instruction in its use.

Work at the individual clinic continues as long as people are waiting to be treated—or until darkness intervenes. In one two-day period 1,000 people turned up. Some were asked to come to the next stopping place.

Figures indicate that 54 per cent of the Negro children under twelve in the county are suffering from malnutrition. A large percentage of the ailments of the adults probably have the same cause. All this is the result of the classical "three M" diet of the southern Negro: meal, meat, and molasses. He buys the cheapest food the commissary affords. Thus there is the paradox of men starving on some of the earth's richest land.

All the lecturing in the world about the value of minerals and vitamins cannot remedy this situation. Protective foods are beyond the pocketbooks of a Negro population such as that of Bolivar, where 20 per cent of families are without any cash income at all. They must either be given these foods free, or taught to raise them. Alpha Kappa Alpha is attempting to strike midway between these two courses.

From the Surplus Commodities Corporation it gets foods to distribute free. Educational work on the value of gardens is also done.

Getting planters to allot space for kitchen gardens and persuading the Negroes to plant them is difficult. Four years is the usual time required to educate a man to raise a garden. By creating an appetite for new foods, the group hopes to cut this time down.

These self-sacrificing women have done an enormous amount of good. They furnish personal contact which is an essential complement to the wide-scale educational work done by Rosenwald, the anti-malaria campaign of WPA, and the syphilis drive put on by the U.S. Public Health Service. This fact is appreciated by alert planters. The group has been invited to other states.

Locally, the impact of their vigorous effort is profound. Large Negro attendance at free syphilis clinics is due for the most part to Alpha Kappa Alpha work. A fraternal organization in the town of Mound Bayou, now health-conscious, dropped plans to build an office building. Funds earmarked for this purpose are going to build a 50-bed hospital. A health insurance plan is also under way.

For her part, Dr. Ferebee feels amply repaid for all her effort when a child who was weak and spindly returns well and healthy for a check-up the next year.

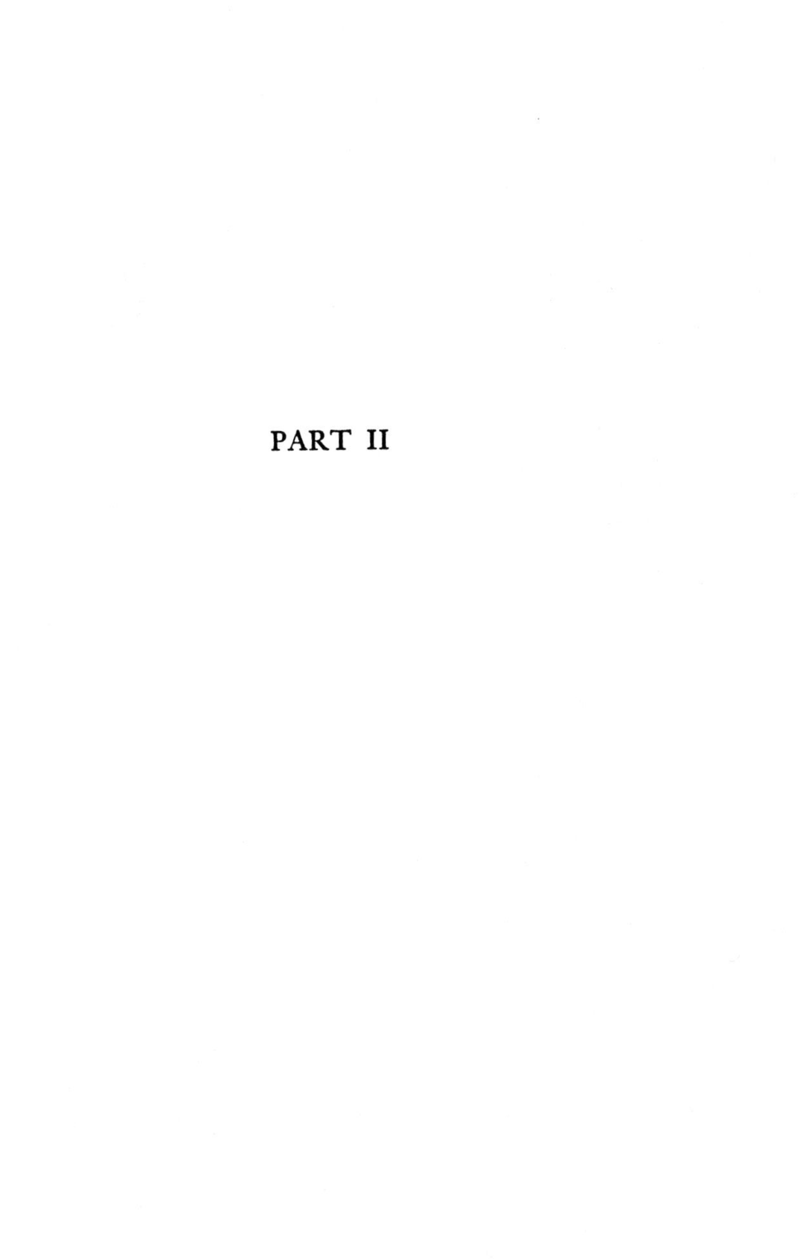

PART II

CHAPTER XVI

SCIENCE PROPHET

At least 90 per cent of the time research work follows a pattern of deadly monotony, patiently plodding a weary path toward a given goal—and sometimes it triumphs.

But there is always the alluring chance that a happy accident may make a short cut across the years—that the worker may blunder upon a fact which opens up entirely new fields. These are the fascinating cases—the sweepstakes winners of research. Luck has forever been the fickle and elusive ally of the research man.

The discovery of synthetic indigo, most widely used of all dyes, is a case in point. For years chemists sought a cheap substitute for the coloring material extracted from plants grown in India and elsewhere. Then one day a worker was stirring a simmering pot of chemicals with a thermometer. He wanted to keep an accurate temperature record. Heat cracked the thermometer, spilling mercury into the chemical stew. Contents of the pot were instantly changed into a beautiful dark blue! Mercury was the catalyst needed for oxidizing naphthalene—for making synthetic indigo!

Every textbook tells how Watt observed the lifting of a teapot lid and used the phenomenon as a basis for his steam engine; how Galileo derived the laws of the pendulum from chance observation of a swaying chandelier; and how Newton saw a falling apple and discovered the earth's gravitational pull on the moon. These stories may be doubtful, but modern science affords a host of examples about which there is no doubt. Such as the discovery of saccharin.

Remsen and Fahlberg were working on some routine chemistry problems at Johns Hopkins, with no thoughts whatsoever of finding a sugar substitute. But one day at lunch Fahlberg noted that his sandwiches were sickeningly sweet. Since when had they started putting sugar in bread, he wanted to know. He took another exploratory bite. This one was all right. Puzzled, he touched his tongue to his fingers. Although he had scrubbed his hands thoroughly, they seemed to be covered with an invisible powder, sweeter than any sugar!

He hurried back to the lab; began searching the beakers with which he had been working. In one of them he found the coal-tar derivative saccharin. The substance, 280 times as sweet as cane sugar, is valuable for diabetics and reducers. Its discovery was pure accident.

Then there was the lecture that Elihu Thomson, who later was to win fame for his work in electricity, gave one day to his chemistry class at Central High School in Philadelphia. Students, unaware that history was about to be made, watched with casual interest while he rapidly whirled a bottle half-filled with liquid. They saw that the centrifugal forces pulled the liquid up the side of the bottle. But they did not see something else that Dr. Thomson was watching excitedly.

By mischance the liquid in the bottle contained some sediment. What amazed Thomson was that the whirling forces separated this sediment from the liquid. Why couldn't this principle be used to separate substances of differing densities? It could. There were scores of applications. The cream separator resulted; and so did the centrifuges used to clarify glues, varnishes and serums. Luck again!

One of the nicest examples of the intervention of luck occurred a few years ago in the General Electric Laboratory. Two workers, McArthur and Eldridge, were investigating problems of short-wave broadcasting. Day after day, while they tinkered with a new high-frequency tube, they complained of headaches and the usual feverish symptoms of the common cold. Dr. Willis Whitney, director of the lab at the time, investigated. While the tube was turned on he noted that body temperature of the men near it rose to 102!

Whitney's head buzzed with the excitement of this thing. He called in Dr. Charles M. Carpenter, a medical man, and they went over it together. In the first place, what was fever? Simply an effort of the body to throw off infection. They knew that Julius Wagner-Jauregg in Vienna had treated paresis patients by deliberately infecting them with malaria. The malaria-induced fever sometimes killed the heat-sensitive syphilis microbe. The idea worked well in many cases. In others death resulted.

Wouldn't an *artificial* fever that could be perfectly controlled get better results, Dr. Whitney asked? Tubes were built into cabinets which would shoot warming waves through a sick man. Temperatures could be lifted as high as 106 and held there for any length of time. A chance observation has opened up a whole new field of healing, valuable in the treatment of a number of diseases.

A leaking can helped Alfred Nobel, Swedish chemist, to perfect dynamite. Nobel was working with nitroglycerine and searching for a way to tame this violent but useful stuff. Nobel's brother had died as the result of a laboratory explosion; other blasts had wrecked trains and ships.

One day the chemist saw that some nitroglycerine had leaked out of a can, spilling onto some sand. A jelly-like stuff resulted which was powerful, yet easy to handle. This was the first crude dynamite.

A similar lucky accident gave Charles Goodyear the secret of vulcanizing rubber. For years he had sought a way to make rubber hard, durable and elastic. Then one day a blob of crude latex and some sulphur slipped from his fingers onto a hot stove. Instantly it was transformed into the substance for which he was looking. On that fortunate accident the modern rubber industry was built.

Anti-knock fuels owe their being largely to the luck factor.

A worker in the General Motors Research Laboratory one day had a crazy hunch: perhaps coloring matter would stop gasoline from knocking. He asked the chemical stock room for materials that might color gasoline. Of the thousands of chemicals on hand the stock keeper happened to pick iodine. It radically reduced knocking properties of gasoline and launched the research which led to the finding of much better substances.

Luck has played a major rôle in the mechanical field. Even the electric meter in your home is there because of an out-and-out accident. Oliver B. Shallenberger, Westinghouse engineer, dropped a small spiral spring into the mechanism of an old-fashioned arc light. It landed in a magnetic field and began to revolve! Here was a perfect measure for electricity.

Hundreds of examples might be cited to show where luck provided us with new comforts, new goods and new weapons against disease. Luck, in fact, provided us with a place to live. Columbus was searching for a route to the East Indies when, quite by accident, he discovered America.

Still the research man who depended on luck alone wouldn't be in business long. The solid fact remains that most triumphs come only after years of patient work. In this section of this book we will see some of this work in the fields of industrial and agricultural research.

It is the medical researcher's job to see that we are not weakened by sickness, destroyed by disease. In a word, he is attempting to present us with extra years of life. The job of the industrial and agricultural researchers is to make that life worth while. They lessen the labor expected of us and provide a more fruitful existence. Few among us are aware of their tremendous influence.

Negligible twenty years ago, industrial research is our fastest-growing profession. This year, alert American manufacturers will spend $180,000,000 in 1,800 laboratories to discover new methods of making their products better and more abundant. In every great industry, research pioneers—mostly anonymous—are devising new twists for the recalcitrant stuffs of nature, extending the frontiers of use and beauty, lowering prices for the consumer, and creating more jobs for labor.

Dr. Karl Compton, president of the Massachusetts Institute of Technology, is perhaps the most articulate spokesman on the subject of industrial research. Let's hear his thoughtful analysis of the way in which it is reshaping our lives.

"Up to now," he states, "mankind has had but two receipts for securing the more abundant life. One was to work hard and long; the other was to take goods from someone else by war, thievery or enslavement.

"The new order of science makes possible for the first time a cooperative creative effort in which everyone is the gainer and no one the loser. Science has the ability to create wealth where wealth did not exist before.

"Since Bell invented the telephone in 1876 the industry has grown into the third largest public utility in the United States, with an investment of nearly five billion and an employment running into hundreds of thousands. Here is a great asset created without taking anything from anybody.

"In America today we see many groups seeking to take things from other groups—by taxation, tariffs, wage scales, unemployment relief, farm subsidies, etc. All these have to do with wealth *distribution*. We do not think intelligently enough in the matter of wealth *creation*, without which schemes of distribution are limited and futile.

"The idea persists that science is a twentieth century dragon. It destroys jobs, creates derelict towns. Such ideas are contrary to fact. They are based on ignorance and misconception, and are vicious in their possible consequences. Yet they have taken an insidious hold on the minds of many people.

"Those who would criticize technological progress have a tremendous job to explain away the continually improving living standards of the American people. Stop to think where we would be if our ancestors had taken steps to impede this movement; and think where oncoming generations will be if we take any foolish action today.

"Fear of research traces to several sources. Some people are upset by the rapid pace of modern life and dread to see anything new. Others think of research in terms of displacement of labor. In thinking of these things it is first necessary to distinguish between two types of research. One is aimed at creating new products, the other at cheapening processes of production of existing products. The first ofttimes produces pure gain in employment. The second can ofttimes achieve the same end if it lowers prices so that larger markets are created.

"Technological unemployment is one of the skeletons in the closet of science. But, frankly, skeletons to me do not seem to be the most important things in the world. We would not advocate abolishing the human race just because it produces skeletons. So let us take a look at this skeleton and try to appraise it honestly.

"A striking example of technological unemployment was given by a recent motor company exhibit. Beside a powerful machine pressing steel wheel parts stood a blacksmith hammering them out by hand. Think of the technological unemployment represented here—thousands of possible blacksmiths replaced by the machine! But think again. Through such developments the modern automobile is made possible at a price within the reach of so many people that it has created an industry which employs one-seventh of all wage earners. This includes those who earn their livelihood by making, distributing and servicing automobiles, or supplying the materials that go into their building, or in the production and sale of oil, or in the building of highways.

"Another similar example comes to mind. Probably the most complete study of the effects of technological improvements on an industry is that of the electric lamp industry conducted by the U.S. Bureau of Labor Statistics. It shows that in the decade 1921–'31 lamp production increased fourfold while man hours of labor employed fell nearly 50 per cent. But what this study did not show was the indirect employment that resulted from lowered costs of electric illumination. Cheaper bulbs meant greater consumption of electricity. This meant new jobs with utilities, in coal mining, in new activities possible at night only because of cheap illumination.

"The whole question can be reduced to a point of absurdity by examining England's textile industry. One hundred years after Watt's invention of the steam engine textile factories used this power and employed 40,000 workers. Had old-fashioned hand looms been employed it would have taken 40,000,000 people to produce the same amount of textiles. Therefore 39,960,000 people were, technically speaking, technologically unemployed. But the population was only 19,-000,000. Thus there were 20,960,000 technologically unemployed unborn babies!

"Let's go back for a moment to the automobile industry. The 1900 census lists 976,000 individuals employed in the wagon industry as manufacturers, drivers, draymen, livery stable employees, blacksmiths, etc. Thirty years later with the advent of the automobile the census lists 2,409,000 individuals engaged in this industry, exclusive of those involved in oil production. They show that while the advent of the automobile created technological unemployment among carriage makers, the net result for labor has been a 250 per cent increase in jobs.

"The chemical industry is one of the best recent examples of the capabilities of the research man. In 1920, there was not a single major chemical company listed on the New York Stock Exchange. For all practical purposes this industry is a creation of the last twenty years. It has been based 100 per cent on scientific research and invention. It is now the third largest industry in the United States and it has in sight still further developments of enormous import.

"About three years ago statistics showed that employment in the chemical industry was 27 per cent higher than in 1929. It is still higher today.

"In individual instances technological unemployment may be a serious social problem—as in a town whose mill has had to shut down or in a craft which has been superseded by a new art. Here the fact that technological unemployment does not exist as measured by overall statistics is of small comfort to families whose wage earners have lost their jobs. Yet this can scarcely be used as an argument against research."

Suppose then, that science has created, rather than destroyed jobs. While working hardships on some people, it has bestowed overall benefits. Do benefits counterbalance hardships? Dr. Compton asks us to look back a few years.

"Just before the advent of the modern machine age the philosopher, John Locke, and the social planner, Jeremy Bentham, were advocating a reorganization of industrial communities so as to utilize the labor of children down to four years of age. This was the only way they could see for increasing productive power so as to raise the standard of living. Now, through science and invention, we have the equivalent of 100 slaves working for each of us in the form of power driven machinery.

"This increased productive capacity has enabled us to decrease the average work week from 60 hours in 1910 to 40 hours at present. Today's wage provides a workman with seven times the goods his wage provided 100 years ago. No amount of legislation, votes or Christian thinking could have accomplished these things.

"We are turning on a good friend indeed when we speak harshly of science. Medicine, sanitation and public health have literally given life to scores of millions of people. Improved agriculture, food technology and transportation have put a quietus on the dismal doctrines of Malthus which held that starvation faced the world after populations reached a certain point."

Convincing as these arguments are, they are unable to talk millions of unemployed workmen out of existence.

"How can we find them jobs? There are several possible moves but the encouragement of scientific research is one of the most important. The forces which, in one lifetime, created the aeronautical, chemical, electrical and automobile industries, can continue to provide new employment.

"To make such a program effective certain obstacles must be overcome. First, I would mention the 'hard-headed, practical business man'; a man without vision, imagination, or enthusiasm for new things; a man whose sole criterion is that to which he has been accustomed. The withering policies of such men have driven many flourishing businesses into obsolescence. In the same class I would place that type of control which focuses attention of profits of the current year to the exclusion of developing strength for the future. Business anemia arises when the cost accountant becomes the master instead of the servant.

"Nothing to me is so disheartening as the industrialist who speaks proudly of the research of his company when, in reality he is supporting a meagre little outfit with only a small fraction of a per cent of his budget. The healthiest companies in the country are spending several per cent of their operating budgets—say five per cent as a good average.

"Several years ago the National Research Council compared the financial standing of industries in relation to their expenditures for research. At the top were the chemical, electrical communications and automobile industries; toward the bottom railroads, lumber and textile industries. The correlation between expenditures for research and financial prosperity was decidedly striking."

Fine for a large, solidly entrenched industry. What about the little fellow?

"There are several ways out for the small industry. It can take its problems to a consulting laboratory. Or, it can take them to the industrial research divisions of educational institutions, or to an organization like the Mellon Institute. An even better approach is for the small industry to hire a man with a good background of chemistry, physics and engineering. One such man with whom I am acquainted saved an oil company thousands of dollars. He noted that temperature fluctuations in oil storage tanks caused "breathing" which expelled thousands of gallons of gasoline into the air. By coating tank exteriors with aluminum he reduced these temperature changes. Saving from this one item alone was sufficient to support an entire research program.

"Patience should be the rule in approaching research problems. Discoveries cannot be made to order for delivery on schedule; and, when made, they cannot be developed overnight into flourishing industries. One should not duplicate the mistake made by a visitor who asked Harvard's President Conant what he was doing in his laboratory. When Conant replied: 'We are seeking to discover the chemical formula for chlorophyl,' his visitor exclaimed: 'Why, how is that? You were working on that problem when I was here last year.'

"Although results may be slow in emerging, past experience has proved this plan to be sure and successful. We can prove that serious general unemployment would have struck us many years earlier had scientific discovery been less encouraged than it was between 1900 and 1930—a period in which twenty million jobs were created.

"When a government official asked me not long ago why science did not have more to offer now, I replied that the groundwork should have been done ten years ago. Similarly, we should now be laying the foundations for ten years hence.

"There is a very great shortage of research men, particularly in chemistry and metallurgy. Even with the notable advances that we have made there are still 150,000 manufacturing concerns which as yet do not support research laboratories. Unfortunately, the number of people that have the particular type of originality required is not large. But for the man who does have real talent this fascinating field presents endless opportunities."

If we accept the fact that science has produced new jobs and new comforts, its closet still contains a very real skeleton. Hasn't science made modern warfare destructive to a point where it threatens the very existence of civilization?

"Admittedly applications of science have enormously increased the horrors and the scope of war. Yet one point should be noted. The lack of science has killed more people and caused more prolonged suffering than all wars in history!

"Insofar as war is caused by natural human cussedness, science can contribute little to helping the situation. Science, per se, is neither good nor bad. It is simply a powerful force which can be used by men for good or evil, depending on their ethical standards and ambitions.

"One of the earliest incentives to war was loot. Later this took the form of control of populations for the purposes of taxation, and exploitation of labor and natural resources. This is all part of the old primitive instinct to secure the good things of life by taking them from someone else. Science has provided a means of gaining the good things without taking them from someone else. To the extent that nations can be induced to support technological development, to that extent can they satisfy their desires without recourse to war.

"Until we arrive at this happy day, science can at least act as a brake on human emotions. I recently saw a cartoon showing two prehistoric cavemen, one armed with a big club, and the other with a primitive bow and arrow. The one with the bow was explaining it as a weapon which would make war so terrible it would end all war. Such arguments only indirectly deter the warlike spirit. Yet a very real horror of war is developing.

"I believe that never before has there been a more nearly universal and sincere desire for peace in the hearts of all people. This was shown by the great reluctance and long delay in the outbreak of the European war despite tensions and provocations which earlier would have led to instant battle.

"Bad as the record of our generation has been, another period was even worse. In the eighteenth century, just prior to the advent of modern science there were only four years in the century without war in Europe. As things stand today the scientist has provided new tools of warfare. How these tools are used is determined not by the scientist alone, but by all of us."

Will science provide a better, happier life in this warless world to come?

"What," asks Dr. Compton, "is happiness? Is it freedom from worry? If that were all the contented cow would epitomize this ideal. We have what the cow has not—imagination, curiosity, ambition, reason and conscience. Science has contributed to these satisfactions. I cannot say whether we are happier in reading news from Europe, or in seeing pictures from Hollywood, or watching a baseball game on Saturday afternoon, than were our forefathers. But I am sure that we now have more avenues for the pursuit of happiness, and shall have even greater ones in the future.

"I cannot predict what the next big developments will be. But they will be important. Among the fields which seem to me to show especial promise: developments of new industrial uses for farm products; improvements in transmission and utilization of electric power; great developments in materials and methods of building construction; increased precision in weather forecasting; a new era in biological discovery; a similar new era in physical science centered around atomic nuclear transformations.

"Our progress may seem slow as we watch and worry day by day, but it is probably a very rapid change in terms of historical perspective."

In the following chapters we will see specifically how individual companies and men are working along the lines suggested by Dr. Compton.

CHAPTER XVII

GLASS MAGIC

Tucked away in the rolling hills of upper New York is the Corning Glass Company. At Corning, the word "research" means two things: first, scientific investigation, in which men spend their lives ferreting out the basic secrets of glass; second, the practical engineering field, where these discoveries are geared to the needs of industry. In vast rambling rooms, amid salt baths and hissing rotary molds, labor 175 scientists. There is singularly little regimentation in the Corning laboratories; to a considerable degree, each man selects some problem that particularly fascinates him and concentrates on it.

Corning's scientists have made glass magnificently versatile. They have fused combinations of sand, soda, lime, borax, lead and other substances to produce over 25,000 variations of glass. They have made glass bolts and nuts, to be used where acids would eat iron. They have made dishes that will not break when filled with molten iron; drinking-glasses that bounce unharmed when dropped on tile floors. Corning has spun filaments so fine that a one-pound batch would stretch around the earth; and has poured the world's biggest chunk of glass—the twenty-ton, 200-inch reflector for the Mt. Palomar telescope.

The gigantic Corning plant itself at first glance resembles a corner of hell. Yet here the raw materials of glass are mixed by laboratory formulas more precise than any medical prescription, and fed into gas-fuelled furnaces. In a cherry-red flood the "cooked" glass spills out into molds; still hot, it is stamped into baking dishes and auto headlights by huge merry-go-round presses. Handworkers fabricate glass so beautiful it is included in museum collections; an automatic machine turns out corrosion-proof insulin ampoules by the million. But whatever the process, whatever the product, it roots inevitably back to research.

Corning always made glass; good glass, judged by traditional standards. Back in 1875, the little company had a line of lamp-chimneys and tubing and "blanks" to be ground into cut-glass vases and bowls. Its industrial research history began in 1908 when Dr. Eugene C. Sullivan was engaged to set up a laboratory. The first problem put before the young scientist was to develop for railway trainmen a lantern globe which wouldn't break in the rain. A brutally tough glass finally emerged.

Few sights are more familiar than the signal lights that gleam along the railroad, the same beautiful red, yellow or green wherever we may be. It was not always so. Years ago, the railroads came to Corning saying, "We have thirty-two shades of green. Some of our yellows look red in murky weather; more dangerous, some of our red lights actually look yellow. Try and straighten this out." Corning determined by test the most readily distinguished red, green and yellow. The resulting color standards were adopted by all American and many foreign railroads.

One day a Corning research man sawed the top off a glass battery jar and ground down its rough edges. That night he took the shallow base home, and asked his wife to bake a cake in it. The improvised baking dish didn't break, and there was excitement in the laboratory next morning. Other researchers began juggling glass formulas and subjecting the product to severe temperatures. Finally, a glass that would resist punishing heat was perfected. Under the name of Pyrex, it has gone into millions of ovens, bringing new beauty to the kitchen and heat-saving efficiency to cooking.

Corning men blew Edison's first light-bulbs in the old-fashioned way, one at a time. When it became apparent that the world wanted bulbs by the billion, research men began to devise machinery to make them better, faster, cheaper. The result is a monstrous engine that goes at too fast a clip to be followed by the eye, producing several hundred bubbles of glass per minute. It has helped reduce the cost of a sixty-watt bulb from $1.75 in 1907 to 15 cents today.

When the World War cut off our supply of technical glassware, imported from Germany, Corning research men set out to develop a new line of beakers, retorts, and test tubes. Eminence in this field got them the job of making one of the most intricate pieces of glass apparatus ever constructed: the perfusion pump of Dr. Alexis Carrel and Charles A. Lindbergh which effectively duplicates the action of the human heart. The country's supply of clinical thermometer-tubing is made at Corning by an ingenious method. Previously, tubing was drawn by hand along a horizontal track. It sagged; quality was uneven. Corning built a 216-foot tower that looks strikingly like the Washington Monument. A chunk of molten glass the size of a punching bag is fixed to the bottom of the tower and a hoist draws it quickly upward. The result is a continuous piece of fine tubing well over 100 feet long. The inside bore is of uniform size—one-third the diameter of a hair.

Corning's new "shrunk" glass is the greatest achievement in glass technology. It is a low-cost duplicate of fused quartz. Fused quartz has been indispensable in the making of various scientific instruments. It is water-clear, permits passage of certain rays that glass stops, and withstands enormously high temperatures. But because it is so costly to melt quartz in electric furnaces, it costs twenty-five times as much as the best glass. In attempting to make a glass to do the same job, Corning research men went through the heartbreak of repeated failures. They tried and abandoned 600 glass formulas. Months passed and the money expended on this dismal daydream mounted to a quarter of a million dollars. The management decided to scrap the project. "Give us a little more time," the scientists begged. They got their reprieve. Like Ehrlich on his magnificent trek through the arsenic compounds which led to the discovery of syphilis-killing 606, they plowed on. Glass No. 790 finally appeared—a material entirely new to the world, 96 per cent pure silica.

Industrialists come to Corning with varied problems. A ginger ale maker, desiring to insure the purity of his product, wanted a glass pipe line running through his factory. The pipe had to be transparent so that he could inspect every inch of it daily, and strong enough to be taken down every night and washed with scalding steam. Corning fabricated a special heat-resistant, shatter-proof glass pipe, now widely used in breweries and in chemical plants.

New problems arise and are disposed of with almost monotonous regularity. Surgeons complain of neck burns from overhead lights in operating rooms. The research men evolve a glass which lets little heat through. Welders want goggles which will cut out eye-damaging light-bands beyond the visible spectrum. The research men oblige. Dr. Chevalier Jackson needed a minuscule light-bulb for his bronchoscope, with which he fishes for foreign objects accidentally sucked down the throat. A bulb no larger than a grain of wheat was designed. Another doctor wanted a glass boot to fit over gangrenous legs; alternate pressure and vacuum inside the boot stimulates blood vessels and hastens mending. Corning came through again, with a contraption which saves many legs from amputation.

The discovery of Steuben glass was a combination of chance and imagination. Medical men wanted a glass for transmission of ultra-violet light. An absolutely new method of glass-making had to be devised in order to make such a material economically possible. After months of experimenting, an unbelievably clear glass, flawless and pure, was produced. Developed for medical science, this super-transparent glass has likewise become a perfect medium for artistic expression. Examples of Steuben glassware have passed the sacred portals of the Victoria and Albert Museum in London and the Metropolitan Museum of Art in New York.

Corning research has developed especially efficient glass insulators for the coast-to-coast telephone line. Conserving electric energy, these insulators have helped to improve the service and bring down the cost of long distance calls. At Berkeley, California, a group of young scientists are experimenting with a huge atom-smasher, called the cyclotron, which has already transformed platinum into gold and has given off more radio-active particles than the world's entire supply of radium. The cyclotron could not function without two insulators of special glass, created by Corning after other materials had failed under heat and the shock of such high voltage. Glass fiber is another proud and very practical Corning achievement. Nearly fifteen times as fine as human hair, this new material, thirty-five million miles of it a year, is being oozed out of invisible nozzles. Some of it is woven into dresses and curtains, some of it into electrical insulation, but most of it goes into the walls of homes.

Splendid achievements, you say, but what effect have they had on employment? Man-hours required to make a piece of plate glass have declined 80 per cent in twenty-five years. Prices have dropped 60 per cent. Increased consumption accompanying lower prices has put 30 per cent more men to work at 50 per cent higher wages. The average annual wage in the glass industry is now $1,300 as against the average in all industries of $1,100. At Corning, during the depression, over three millions were invested in new buildings and equipment; and despite new automatic machinery, employment rose steadily. This is true of glass manufacturing as a whole; in 1939, this 400-million-dollar industry employed 13 per cent more people than in 1929.

Amory Houghton, 40, great-grandson of the Corning founder, son of the former Ambassador to Great Britain, and present head of the business, feels that research should go at an ever-accelerating pace. He sees the glass researcher's skill utilized to build a shiny new world. He foresees houses built of glass bricks and partitioned with glass-bubble slabs which may be sawed and nailed; furnished with glass tables and chairs and draped with glass textiles; equipped with windows which permit light to enter but none to escape—thereby maintaining privacy in a sunlit room. He envisions automobiles insulated with glass wool, using glass spark plugs and running on roads paved with glass blocks; piping and plumbing fixtures made of glass; and a malleable glass which can be worked on machine-shop lathes.

Research scientists are cautious, but even the most conservative say that there is no limit to the future uses of glass; all agree that research in glass will never be concluded. As Corning's veteran research chief, Dr. E. C. Sullivan, puts it: "In glass, not even the easy things have been done. And help is needed for those who like to do the hard things. Tomorrow's better world lies just beyond today's frontiers of research."

CHAPTER XVIII

RESEARCH ODYSSEY

"IN roulette the odds are against you. Play long enough and you always lose. With industrial research the precise opposite is true. Keep at it and you are bound to win." The speaker is Dr. C. E. K. Mees, 59, the amiable, sharp-witted director of Eastman Kodak's huge research department. Proof of his words comes from 29 years' observation.

During this time he has seen research pay off handsomely in the form of home movies, radically improved photo equipment, better plates for astronomers. The whip of money and brains sent researchers off on many devious paths in the magic land of chemistry. They set the company making scores of products, odd to the outsider who thinks of Eastman only in terms of cameras and films. These things touch our everyday lives: artificial silks, wool and leather; vitamins and lacquers; the transparent winding that protects lampshades from dust; and the plastic that goes to make auto steering wheels, flutes, football helmets.

To Dr. Mees, research is the yeast of social change. It provides a more bountiful life for consumers, more profits for the company, more jobs for labor. During the decade 1929–'39 U.S. employment fell 9 per cent. Eastman's rose 75 per cent with $19,000,000 added to payrolls. Two-thirds of the people today employed at the vast Rochester, New York plant are making things which are entirely new or which have been radically improved since 1929.

This company, which has thrived on research was even born of it. A snapshot in the 70's required a horse-drawn cart full of equipment: a dark tent, chemical baths, a bulky camera and sensitizing materials to be applied to wet plates immediately before use. When George Eastman marketed the dry plate he took the horse out of photography. His flexible film made motion pictures possible. When Edison first saw a sample of this film he called his helpers together. "That's it. We've got it. Now work like hell," he enthused.

Eastman has thirteen plants throughout the world, but most activity is centered at 400-acre Kodak Park in Rochester. This is the chief supply center for the 200,000 miles of film consumed annually by the movie industry; and for film needed to make 700,000,000 snapshots taken each year in the United States.

In a sense, the 83 buildings are all materializations of the vapors that rise from test tubes. In one darkened building giant machines roar as they coat emulsion on super quality paper; in another 5 tons of silver per week are dissolved in strong acids—to make photo-sensitive materials. In great halls film packers work in almost complete darkness; some rooms faintly illuminated by a ghostly green glimmer, and others by a pale ruby red.

Air in buildings is humidified and cooled by the world's largest refrigeration plant. Everything is miraculously clean. A fleck of dust on a movie sound track might cause a roar of rage during a tender love scene; or make an unsightly pimple on a photograph. Chimneys as high as 30-story buildings carry smoke away. Switch engines run without fires—every hour or so they are charged with high-pressure steam. Six miles of paved roadway within the park are regularly vacuum cleaned!

All of this is a solid monument to research—research which has made 40,000 jobs, and provided 19,000,000 U.S. camera fans with an inexpensive hobby. It has meant uninterrupted stock dividends since 1902; and wage dividends for workmen totaling over $50,000,000!

Prior to 1912 Eastman's company had done scattered experimental work but had no organized research department. That year he went abroad to hire Dr. Mees, at the time working with a small manufacturer of photographic equipment in England. To get Mees, he had to buy the company. Before the deal was concluded Mees warned his future employer not to expect striking research results for at least ten years. The prediction was astonishingly accurate. Home movies, a product of laboratory research, were introduced in 1923.

At the outset problems presented seemed almost insurmountable. Professional movie cameras cost $500 and weighed 40 pounds. Tripods weighed another 30. Raw film cost 4 cents a foot and a foot lasted one second in a projection machine. Whittling down this bulk and expense was problem No. 1. No. 2 was to find a practical reversal method for finishing; so that one strip of film could act as both negative and positive. Five years of work were required.

The problem of color for home movies came along naturally. Two amateurs, working in New York, had made a promising start. Both were musicians: Leopold Mannes, pianist, and Leopold Godowsky, violinist. Mees invited them to join the research staff. They came, intending to spend a few months, and ended by staying ten years.

But they worked out a marvelously clever process for laying five separate layers of emulsion on movie film: one each for red, yellow and blue with neutral layers of filter between. This was Kodachrome, the color film.

All this work was costly and time-consuming—but it netted business which now totals millions of dollars each year. Thousands of these films arrive at the plant daily to be processed by automatic developing machines. A 15 per cent sampling goes to projection rooms for a check of quality and subject matter—Eastman can't send doubtful material through the mails.

The first World War launched a chain of investigation that paid off handsomely. The sensitizing dyes will illustrate.

Films made by ordinary procedures are sensitive only to blue-violet light. Reds and yellows photograph as black. But when sensitizing dyes are added you get a panchromatic film; a film, that is, sensitive to all color shadings. Germans had discovered the only dyes available for this purpose; yet Mees felt that others existed. Several times he was on the point of abandoning the expensive eight-year search. "I was scared stiff to go on, and frightened to death to stop," he says. He let the second fear prevail.

In the end Eastman chemists discovered scores of new dyes, better than any known before. Panchromatic films made from them produced finer snapshots; and banished the old ailment of the movie industry, klieg eyes. This temporary blindness was caused by ultra-violet radiation from arc lamps. When it was possible to substitute yellow light from tungsten bulbs for the blue from arc lamps cases of eyestrain ended.

The first World War similarly launched Eastman on another research project. In 1914, German supplies of organic chemicals, needed for laboratory research, were cut off. Research everywhere was endangered. Mees tried to get others to stock the huge range of exotic chemicals needed. They refused. He took his story to Eastman, proposing that the company take on the job. "How much will we lose?" his employer asked. Mees said at least $100,000. Eastman said to go ahead. Today there are 3,300 organics in the list. The strangest one: a synthetic skunk scent—valuable for alarm systems in mines. Men working underground with noisy machinery can't hear bells, but they can smell powerful skunk odor wafted through the mine by ventilating fans. The organics represent a profitable sideline; and they remove the danger of U.S. research suffering a shut-down because of events happening elsewhere in the world.

Dr. Mees' interests are as varied as the products of his laboratory. He is an amateur Egyptologist. Several years ago he decided to learn Russian—and did, with the aid of a

Rochester streetcar conductor born in that country. He likes his research men to have similarly limber minds. With salty humor, he insists that they be given complete freedom. "The man who knows most about any project," he says, "is the man doing the job. The man immediately above him knows a little less about it, and the research director considerably less. By the time you get up to a committee of vice-presidents they know precisely nothing."

The work of Dr. Kenneth Hickman shows how this policy of freedom can produce results valuable to company and public alike.

Hickman, a capable, enthusiastic young Englishman was working with vacuum pumps and molecular stills; looking particularly for any applications they might have to problems of film drying. In principle, the molecular still is very much like old-fashioned stills used to make whisky, gasoline and turpentine. But there is one important difference.

In ordinary stills molecules swarm off a heated surface like so many angry bees, colliding with each other and with molecules of air. A molecular still works under high vacuum. This allows individual molecules to travel in a straight and unobstructed path from the heated surface to the cooled surface where they are condensed.

Chemists had frequently used molecular stills made of metal—with discouraging results. Their notebook calculations would predict a certain set of reactions, then quite a different set would take place. So Hickman decided to make his stills of glass. Then he could *see* what was happening.

Fascinated, he hovered over them while molecules by the billion hopped across the gap to condense as visible liquids. Molecules took on personalities. British-wise, he was soon calling them "chaps."

It was a long intellectual leap from this pure science to practical results; from swarming molecules to vitamins which would prevent bone-bending rickets, and vitamins to cure the muscular dystrophy which cripples so many older people. Hickman made this leap one hot July afternoon.

He was walking down a Rochester street and paused to look into a sun-drenched drugstore window. Wasn't the sun destroying vitamins in the cod liver oil displayed there? Wouldn't it be better if those vitamins were concentrated, thereby becoming more stable? Now in the molecular still . . .

Hickman didn't know that a research man in England was having approximately the same thoughts at about the same time. But this is of no importance here. The point is that neither fish oils nor vegetable oils had ever been distilled before. They were "fixed" fats. One research group had spent half a million dollars trying to refine linseed oil in ordinary stills. The effort was a dead loss.

Chemically speaking, a miracle happened when Hickman put cod liver oil in his glistening glass still. The oil began to break down! Globules of a waxy fat collected on the condenser. Hickman, in his notebook, called these globules "a concentration of therapeutically valuable substances." This meant that he didn't know what he had. But assay by a pharmaceutical house indicated it to be one of the best vitamin concentrates ever made. It was potent and all but tasteless. Together with General Mills, Eastman set up a new company to make vitamins A, C, D and E. This company, launched by a lucky research break, is the world's largest maker of Vitamin A concentrate. It buys oils—from cod, tuna, shark, halibut and dogfish—by the tankcar and markets vitamins by the ton.

This research sideline, even had its own sideline! Better pumps were needed to exhaust air from stills. Hickman built them—the most efficient commercial pumps ever made. They had hundreds of applications elsewhere: in making better X-ray, television and radio broadcasting tubes.

Research, likewise, led Eastman far off the photographic

track in its plant at Kingsport, Tenn. This branch was originally set up to cut timber from 40,000 acres of leased land and convert it into wood alcohol—needed as a solvent for film base. When others discovered how to make wood alcohol synthetically the plant lost much of its usefulness. Then research men had another idea. The disastrous fire of X-ray film which killed 124 people at the Cleveland Clinic in 1929, plus the rapid growth of the home movie industry, made development of safety film imperative. Kingsport was an obvious place for production of this product, cellulose acetate, because of a readily available supply of cotton.

Research men, never content, asked what else might be done with cellulose acetate. They have given a steady stream of answers: artificial silks—including a rich new crepe—wrapping materials similar to cellophane, transparent sheeting used for cake covers and flower boxes, plastics—and even a charcoal briquette used on railway diners! As a result of research effort $17,000,000 worth of these products are being sold each year; and jobs have been made for 6,000 people!

Fortuitously, the research men have just produced a radically new optical glass. It is unlike any glass ever before produced. Instead of being made of silica—sand—it is composed almost entirely of rare elements: thorium, boron, tungsten, barium, lanthanum. The search for this glass took seven years. When told of the patent application at Berlin, German technicians were incredulous. Hadn't they tried and failed to produce such a glass? With Teutonic stolidness they refused to believe in its existence—even after they had seen samples!

The new Eastman miniature camera—the $300 Ektra—likewise arrived at a propitious moment. Five years of work went into its development. The job was completed just as supplies of the German Leica and Contax were threatened.

Eastman has paid a staggering price for its research. Personnel has grown from twelve men in 1912 to 400 today; and annual expenditures for experimental work from $50,000 to

$5,000,000. Expenditures for research now run about 25 cents for every dollar earned. Facilities provided the research man are as magnificent as any on earth. If a man wants to try a new movie film, he has a complete Hollywood set—and even a 180-seat theatre. He has the world's largest library of photographic literature at his command and nearly every other facility that can be imagined.

Cost? "If you hit something really good," says Dr. Mees, "the research cost is insignificant. And if you don't—well, why cry over spilt milk?" Then he pointedly adds: "I've never yet heard of a company going bankrupt because it spent too much on research."

Before him he sees a vast mass of work to be done. He wants color for amateur snapshots and more fundamental facts about the theory of photography. He looks on the latter as a vast mosaic with at least half the pieces missing.

Continued healthy growth of the industry depends on this search. "Perhaps it was once true that if you built a better mousetrap the world would make a path to your door," he says. "But today your competitor will think up a still better mousetrap, hire Charlie McCarthy to advertise it on the radio and drive you out of business."

CHAPTER XIX

MAN WITH A MILLION IDEAS

INDUSTRIAL research has its lone wolves, as well as its great company-owned laboratories. These men tinker for their own amusement and profit. Occasionally they happen on something good, but sustained production is rare among them. Carleton Ellis was a glowing exception to this rule. At the time of his death a year ago he held more patents than any living man—810.

We live constantly with his works. When we arise in the morning we scrub our teeth with liquid dentifrices, drink from unbreakable tumblers, and wash with soaps which trace to his thinking. Our breakfast cream comes in bottles protected by waxed hoods of his devising, our eggs are fried in his vegetable fats and we eat off tables covered with his lacquers. Possibly the flowers on the table were grown in a chemical fertilizer of his making. We start our cars by pulling a choke button made of one of his plastics and drive on gasoline made under his patents. So it goes throughout the day.

The tall, slender, grey-haired inventor lived and worked at Morristown, New Jersey. He had deep-set studious eyes and a thought-wrinkled brow. One is naturally tempted to draw parallels between Ellis and Edison. Both produced prodigiously; and both managed with only a few hours' sleep each night. Points of similarity end here. Edison's formal education totaled three months in public school at Port Huron, Michigan; Ellis graduated at the Massachusetts Institute of Technology. Edison experienced years of grinding poverty; Ellis was an immediate success.

Ellis's patents made several million dollars; built the inventor homes in Montclair, on Cape Cod, and in Nassau. Always, he was alone; a man who conceived a new product, worked out technical details and then sold the patent to the highest bidder. His life was a vastly exciting adventure with ideas.

Weaving his way through the difficult field of chemistry, this versatile genius produced new paints, lacquers, resins. He developed the oil-cracking process under which Standard Oil of New Jersey has produced 40 *billion* gallons of gasoline; and the process to make vegetable oils into fluffy cooking fats like Crisco.

For two years after graduation from M.I.T., Ellis stayed on as an instructor. It was during this period that he got the spark which set him off on his life work.

One day he watched a workman remove paint from a piece of furniture. First he softened the paint with wood alcohol. When this was scraped off the wood was left a dirty, stained brown. Next, the painter bleached it white with oxalic acid.

Most people wouldn't have given the matter a second thought. It annoyed Ellis. All that tedious, time-consuming work simply to remove a thin layer of paint! Why, there should be a solvent to do the job quickly, and in one operation. There should be, and there probably was, if someone would only take the time to find it. Ellis proposed to take the time.

Between classes and lectures, and during hours when most sensible people were sleeping, he worked in a chemistry lab with smelly solvents that bit at his nostrils. He'd paint them on boards covered with hard, ancient paint. At times the solvents were strong enough to dissolve board as well as paint. Other times they stained the wood; or bubbled into a gooey mess.

Finally he hit upon a mixture of alcohol, benzol and paraffin, which did the complete job in one operation. Ellis borrowed $500, rented a shed in a suburb of Boston and started marketing his patented paint remover by door-to-door sales. The business blossomed into an overnight success when the Pennsylvania Railroad placed a $5,000 order—for an entire carload. On the strength of this he gave up teaching.

Ellis heard that there was difficulty in soldering a new metal just coming into commerce—aluminum. A flux was needed to make solder and aluminum stick together. A small problem, perhaps, but one that had to be solved if the silvery metal were to gain an important place in industry. With solder, soldering iron, and sheet aluminum he went to work. Three weeks later he had the needed flux.

A large part of this desire to create new products traced to impatience with the world as it existed. People were altogether too prone to accept things as perfect simply because they were familiar. Ellis, on the other hand, was painfully aware of the imperfections which he wished to correct.

In partnership with Nathaniel Foster, lawyer, he set up his own laboratory at Larchmont, New York. How was this quiet, rather unassuming man able to range over so much territory? Where, indeed, does the difference lie between an inventive nut tinkering in an attic, and a man who made millions dealing in things as ephemeral as ideas?

"Three things," said Ellis, "are necessary to success. Business ability and willingness to work are quite as important as a capacious imagination. The successful inventor must be a gambler to the extent that he will plunge into new territory with hope alone as his guide. At the next moment he must go about the relatively monotonous business of straightening a wrinkle from some industrial process."

In 1909, Ellis launched his attack on the petroleum molecule. When he began work, oil distilled in simple pot stills yielded less than 40 per cent gasoline. Heavier fuels such as kerosene were piling up at an alarming rate. Ellis foresaw that an expanding auto industry was going to create a market for huge quantities of gasoline. More of this fuel had to be squeezed from petroleum.

Somehow he had to crack the petroleum molecule and fit the pieces together again in a new pattern to make gasoline. In other words, make more gasoline out of a barrel of crude. Using temperatures and pressures almost unheard of in industry at the time, Ellis developed his "tube and tank" method of cracking. One hundred gallons of good crude were made to yield as much as 90 gallons of gasoline! Standard Oil of New Jersey operates under these patents.

Study of the fascinating hydrocarbons in crude oil yielded more ground to the prying Ellis mind. He found a means of extracting iso-propyl alcohol from refinery wastes. At the time it was a chemical curiosity selling for $5 a gram. Today it costs less than $1 a gallon and is the basis for most rubbing alcohols; and for Vapon, a "dry" shampoo.

These jobs represent work in the rarefied upper atmosphere of chemistry: a place where Ellis spent much of his time. But he wasn't above coming down to earth on occasion. Take the case of the dog biscuit. A packing house owner presented this problem.

Could anything, he wanted to know, be done with milk left in udders of slaughtered cows? Sanitary laws prohibited its use as human food. Was there anything against using it as dog food, asked Ellis? Not that he knew of, said the packer.

Ellis knew nothing about cookery so he took a night off to read up on it. Propped up in bed he read half a dozen books on animal diet and culled a few recipes for making biscuits and cakes. Next morning he had a biscuit board, an oven, cooky cutters and other assorted paraphernalia delivered to the lab. He mixed the refuse milk, bran and other substances into a batter which he rolled and baked. A dog sniffed at the biscuits, took an exploratory bite and then left them severely alone.

Then Ellis had a hunch. Perhaps a biscuit shaped like a bone would be more tempting to choosy canine appetites.

With shears he snipped out a special bone-shaped cutter. Dogs ate these biscuits readily! Why? Even after making upwards of $100,000 from this patent, Ellis still didn't know.

Naturally all of the thousands of ideas developed weren't successful. Ellis thought that a synthetic resin might be substituted for chicle in chewing gum. He issued orders for the lab staff to chew all new resins developed. Dental bills rose alarmingly and some of the resins had to be pried out of teeth with screw drivers. Eventually a fairly satisfactory resin was found. It wasn't good enough to displace chicle in better chewing gums, but was all right for the penny blobs bought by children.

The laboratory's achievements in the first World War are well known. Chemical warfare men broadcast an appeal to all chemists to get busy on the problem of acetone production. This material was needed in huge quantities as a solvent for the "dope" used on airplane wings.

Ellis replied within a few days. He had found a ready source of supply. Army men, frankly incredulous, hurried to the lab. While they watched, Ellis made a gallon of the stuff, using only laboratory equipment. Then he explained how he had completed the job so quickly. While doing some work with waste gases from oil refineries, he discovered a way to extract acetone. At the time, the process had seemed valueless, since there was little use for the colorless, aromatic solvent. But when the demand arose, he simply turned back to the voluminous notes kept on all work. There he found all the details. Within a few weeks of this demonstration acetone was being produced in tankcar lots!

His sorcery extracted a host of other things from petroleum: a fat substitute, valuable in soap making; synthetic resins; and even a butter substitute.

One of the outstanding Ellis jobs was production of edible fats from cottonseed, peanut, coconut and other vegetable oils. Millions of gallons of these oils were available, but

American housewives were accustomed to using lard in cooking. How could the oils be converted into a solid fat, something that looked like, and had the properties of, lard?

Ellis reviewed the chemistry of the situation. There was room in each of the oil molecules for another atom of hydrogen. Ellis worked for months finding how to attach this extra atom. Under various conditions he bubbled the gas through cottonseed oil. One day he produced a miniature snowstorm! Flakes of solid white fat began to form! When chilled and pressed these flakes turned out to be an excellent fat.

Crisco and similar substances trace largely to this work. The chief significance of this discovery: any country with an adequate supply of vegetable oils would never again have to face a fat shortage such as threatened the United States during the last war.

On one trip to Germany Ellis carried along letters of introduction—just as Lindbergh carried them on his flight to Paris. German chemists who received them roared with laughter. Hadn't they read Ellis's eight books, at least two of which were bibles in their field? And hadn't they read his contributions to chemical literature, and followed his amazing patent saga?

Ellis was born in Keene, New Hampshire; had much the same life as any active boy born to parents in modest circumstances. His youth produced no anecdotes to serve as clues to genius, but he did have a sharply developed business sense.

As a youngster Ellis was given a camera and spent thirty painfully accumulated dollars buying supplies to make his own plates. This, according to his foundryman father, was a sheer waste of good money. The boy set about proving his better judgment. He knew his New England neighbors well enough to realize that they would hesitate about paying to have their pictures taken. So he toured the countryside asking permission of farmers to photograph their horses. Flattered, the horse owner would sidle into the picture. Nearly always he wanted to buy a print.

In recent years the plastics field was the chief Ellis love. His laboratory produced upwards of 100,000 synthetic resins. The vast majority were hopelessly bad, a few promising, and perhaps a dozen or so really good. Two of these good ones are bases for quick-drying lacquers—products which helped revolutionize the auto industry by making painting a job to be reckoned in hours, rather than in weeks.

Travel always stimulated Ellis. One of his most successful ideas came while he was vacationing with his wife in Germany, during the summer of 1922. He was visiting the vast German chemical trust, I. G. Farbenindustrie. A guide pointed to enormous stock piles of sugary-looking urea. Production of the stuff, the guide sadly explained, far exceeded demand. Perhaps Herr Ellis had an idea?

Ellis had no idea at the moment but he lost no time getting one when he was back in his own laboratory. Urea should, he thought, be an ideal base for plastics. For months he ground away at the problem. Finally he came up with a milk-white, ivory-like substance, unlike any of its predecessors in the field. The material had magnificent possibilities. Since it was white (rather than dark brown like most plastics) it could be dyed any color. Ellis enthused about possibilities. Why, it could be used for jewelry, tableware, lampshades, pens, dressing-table fittings, radio cabinets . . .

It is dangerous business for an inventor to project his ideas and hopes too far into the future. But Ellis's enthusiasm was justified. It did indeed find a thousand uses. One company alone employs 250 men to make 12,000,000 pounds per year of this urea plastic.

Ellis picked up other ideas on his travels. On a trip to Arizona, in 1934, he noted the hard, bitter, wild-growing jojoba nuts. A few of the poorer natives roasted and ground them into a tasteless substitute for coffee. Other possibilities?

Ellis sent a few bushels back to the laboratory; got busy on them when he returned. From them he extracted an ingredient for a linoleum-like floor-covering, and a filler for quick-drying inks, necessary in modern high-speed printing.

It is impossible to estimate how many thousands of jobs trace to his work. There is hardly a branch of the huge chemical industry that doesn't link to it in some way.

———   ———   ———

Bill Clapp is a happy-go-lucky contrast to Ellis; a man who has picked a quiet research corner all his own and stayed contentedly in it. He has spent the better part of his life studying a very special kind of worm; a fragile marine animal so delicate that it all but defies handling by human hands. Yet this creature is sturdy and persistent enough to honeycomb the toughest woods: teak, mahogany and eucalpytus. This is the teredo. It looks like a grey-white worm, but is actually a mollusk, a relative of the oyster and clam.

The destruction caused by these termites of the sea is mighty to behold. They eat through ropes to cut yachts adrift, and destroy planking in boats. In one four-year invasion of San Francisco Bay they destroyed $25,000,000 worth of property, and did upwards of $5,000,000 damage in Boston Harbor in three years. They now appear to be ready to attack the world's biggest, richest harbor: New York.

Generally speaking, marine borers fall into two large classifications: the Mollusca, which are relatives of the clam; and the Crustacea, which are kin of the crabs, shrimps and lobsters. There are thousands of individual members of these destructive clans, but their minor points of difference are interesting only to the marine biologist. To the owner of property which touches salt water the performance of all of them is the same. They rasp their way into wooden piling, leaving no visible mark of entrance on the outside.

A pile which looks thoroughly sound may contain tens of thousands of borers, some of which are as much as 6 feet long!

The intricate weaving of their tunnels, which never cross, may give the interior of an oak timber the cross-section appearance of a piece of molasses candy. In such a condition its structural strength is zero. Timbers which look virginally sound, may be broken over the knee.

The world center for research with these dangerously destructive pests is a laboratory as unusual as the borers themselves. It is housed in a barn and exists without any subsidies. It sends no bills. If clients, which include oil, railroad, and steamship companies, are satisfied with work done for them they judge the value of service rendered and send checks accordingly. As a possible commentary on human nature, note in passing that the laboratory always totters uncomfortably on the verge of bankruptcy. Yet William F. Clapp will have things no other way.

"Friends are always attempting to make me change my ways," says this genial biologist. "They want me to keep books and send bills and do things like that. But I'm damned if I will. I am a biologist, not a bookkeeper."

If a check arrives and Clapp feels that he has not earned the sum sent, he returns it. A large sugar company called for advice about a new dock. A telephone call saved them thousands of dollars and they sent a $500 check in appreciation. Clapp returned it. No five minute telephone call could be worth that much, he contended. Another time he refused an annual retainer of $15,000 from a company which made a wood preservative.

As highly unorthodox as all this is, everything works agreeably in the small barn laboratory which sits beside Duxbury Bay on the Massachusetts coast. Whenever anything is really needed it seems to appear; whether it be a compound microscope, a pressure treater for applying experimental woods preservers, or a new filing cabinet. A railroad company official noted that the laboratory was so cold one winter that workers found it necessary to wear overcoats. A few days later a check for $1,000—enough for a new steamheating system—arrived.

Clapp, 60, is chunky, sandy-haired. He has a pleasant toothy grin and an engaging manner. He has been on the faculties of both Harvard and the Massachusetts Institute of Technology, and is one of the founders of the new science of biological engineering. Despite this impressive academic background, he has no degree. In college he took only courses which interested him, rather than ones leading to a degree.

This inclination to follow natural interests probably accounts for the pleasantly informal set-up of the Clapp laboratory. The seven people who work there—at $25 a week—eat at the generous table provided by Mrs. Clapp; and all live in the large, rambling house which is a hundred or so yards from the laboratory. There is little of the musty ceremony of science about this enthusiastic group of young researchers. They play in a rummy tournament that by now has become a house tradition, have an occasional cocktail at the country inn across the road from the laboratory, and discuss marine borers with the same vehemence that other people discuss politics.

Although the laboratory concerns itself with anything that causes deterioration of structural materials, it is primarily concerned with the ravages of marine borers which, in an average year, do $50,000,000 worth of damage along the U.S. coast.

Of all the borers, Teredo navalis is the most interesting. He is a swift, dramatic performer. He brings docks crashing down and can completely destroy a costly wharf in as little as two months. He is the shipworm of the ancients. Greek and Roman navies sheathed their fighting ships with copper to save them from his ravages, and the U.S. Army recently spent $2,000,000 repairing its Boston docks which had received his attentions. Let's see something of this impressive creature.

He is launched into the world as a free-swimming larva, minute in size but immensely promising. He is the product of a sexual relationship as casual as any in the world. His mother, living chastely in her own burrow, deposits her eggs and holds them in her gill chamber. Presently sperm, discharged into the water by some isolated male, is drawn into her body and flushed through her gill chamber. A good proportion of her 500,000 eggs are thus fertilized. Eggs are held in the body for hatching and launched only when conditions are favorable for development. They may wait out the winter in the embryonic state before emerging as a purplish cloud. From this moment onward, each individual is on his own.

Sea currents deposit some of them on rocks, some on the mud bottom, and some on wooden piling. Wherever they land they instantly answer some urge of instinct and start burrowing. Those that landed on mud and rock quickly perish. Those that alight on timber are more fortunate. After two hours of furious work their minute heads, shaped like clam shells, have rasped away a shelter deep enough to enclose the entire body.

As he progresses from the embryonic to the adult stage, teredo becomes a rather complex and impressive creature. He sheds his fragile shell with which he does his boring and gets another which is more sturdy. He develops stomach, intestines, heart, kidneys and a simple but satisfactory nervous system. He is now ready to do real damage.

Teredo maintains contact with the outside world, which is to say the sea, by two hair-like branches of a forked tail. Through one he sucks in sea water—and food in the form of minute sea life—and through the other exhausts his body wastes. The opening through which these two siphons extend is no larger than a pinhead, but this portal will serve teredo even though his body attains a length of two feet. It acts as a superbly constructed valve. The tail can be manipulated to close the burrow whenever danger approaches—danger in the form of jellyfish, oil, or polluted water. Teredo can survive for several weeks in the security of his tightly locked home.

Teredo is a master architect and a superb housekeeper. He

allows no waste or litter to accumulate in his tunnel. He removes all débris by the only means at his disposal—by eating it. He lines his tunnel neatly with lime. At danger spots—where another creature may be attempting to cut a path through his domain—the teredo will secrete a thick wall of lime. In some cases this tunnel is so thick and hard that it cannot be broken by the strongest fingers.

In most cases these borers will construct only enough tunnel to accommodate their bodies, although there must be a slight excess space to accommodate for building errors. Perhaps the rasping head will get dangerously near a crack in the wood. In this case the borer must have room to squeeze his body back into the tunnel and go off in a safer direction.

His burrow may approach those belonging to other members of his kind, but they never cross. Perhaps only a membrane of wood will separate them but each will maintain its discreet identity. The teredo may bore directly through a timber but he will never bore through to the open on the side opposite his entrance. Something warns him that he is approaching the open—and destruction—and he will change the course of his tunnel.

When the constant rocking motion of his head has worn out a set of denticles—or teeth—teredo sprouts another. As many as a hundred rows of these microscopic teeth have been found in one of these creatures. Fragile as they are, no structural wood has yet been found, which is dense enough to resist their boring action. Some varieties of teredo can even cut their way through poorly mixed concrete.

Whether the sawdust he consumes is utilized as food is a matter of dispute. Most authorities think that it is, but Clapp doesn't agree. He maintains that Teredo's boring is simply an adventure in home building, and that he subsists on plankton, the microscopic drifting life of the seas. Temperature of water determines the span of each year's activity: in Boston it is two months; in the tropics the teredo works the year around. An untreated timber which would last 30 years in Labrador, may last only one year in Panama.

Why will borers suddenly invade a harbor which has gone unmolested for decades? The answer usually lies in changed conditions. A three-year drought explained the infestation at San Francisco. With very little fresh water going into the Bay, salinity rose and the borers went to work to do staggering damage. Particular attention is now being centered on New York Harbor. In the past, pollution of this port has been so great that borers could not exist. When the present clean-up program is completed, they will almost surely arrive in large numbers and go to work. Such a thing happened at Lynn, Massachusetts, and elsewhere.

Keeping track of borer activity in a hundred harbors scattered throughout the Western Hemisphere is the monumental task the Clapp Laboratory has cut out for itself. Are borers on the increase in Puerto Rico? And what varieties are at work in New Brunswick? Harmless ones which work in water too deep to damage piling, or the destructive Limnoria? To answer such questions Clapp's endlessly active mind has devised many ingenious aids. He has constructed a test block which gives a continuous record of borer activity, and a trap which captures specimens for identification.

The test block is engaging in its simplicity. It consists of nine small blocks of pine—ideal teredo fodder—bolted to a strap of iron. Each month one block is removed, and a new one is bolted in its place. Biologists examine the block in the laboratory and compare it with those removed from the same spot at earlier dates. They can thus determine whether borer population is rising or falling.

The teredo traps consist of 30 shingles bolted together. Since the borers refuse to cross a crack, they confine activity to a single shingle. When the bundle is unbolted whole specimens may be removed, examined, identified.

Test boards are kept at over 400 stations, and traps at scores of others. Maintenance of a board costs about $5 a month and a few companies pay for this service, but the great burden of expense falls on the laboratory. Test boards occasionally reveal a tremendous upsurge of borer population. In severe cases as many as 100 teredos have been found boring in a single square inch of wood! Such cases demand instant attention. Several times Clapp has found it expedient to wire dock owners to quickly remove all valuable goods from their property; that their docks were in danger of collapse.

Once test boards indicate that borers are at work on the piling which supports a large dock, a diver goes down to make an examination. Some of the divers that work for Clapp are so skilled that they even know Latin names of the most prevalent borers. With astonishing accuracy they can estimate the structural strength of supporting material under the dock.

Corrective measures are determined by local conditions. Where damage is severe piling must be replaced. Sometimes concrete corsets are poured around partially damaged piling, and other times they are covered with metal sheathing. Damage to the vast $25,000,000 Army Base in Boston was so severe that Clapp recommended that bulkheads be built which would completely enclose the sub-structure of the dock; and that fill be pumped in. This fill prevented further activity of the borers, since ready access to salt water is necessary for their existence.

If timbers in new construction are pressure treated with good quality creosote they get complete protection. But in some cases the quality of creosote is so low and method of application so bad that even this treatment is valueless. The Clapp Laboratory tests protective power of these materials. Through ignorance or false economy, hundreds of thousands of untreated piles are still being used in U.S. harbors. As a result docks only last a third as long as they should.

At least one favorable thing may be said for marine borers: without them the world would have no harbors. Long ago they would have been choked by rotting driftwood, and trees brought down to the sea by rivers. By eating this débris the borers have kept them open to the sea.

Clapp's haphazardly run little laboratory was founded in 1933. Prior to this he conducted his researches aboard a sailing ship which friends bought for him. Before he converted the ship into a marine biological laboratory, it had worked the New England coastal trade, and had helped carry granite from Maine to build the Washington Monument.

When the 60-year-old schooner sank in Duxbury Bay in 1933, Clapp moved equipment into the barn which houses the laboratory at present. The information stored in this ancient structure is astonishing in scope. Its collection of marine borers is greater than that owned by all museums in the world. It keeps individual records of a third of a million piles, and has detailed information on borer activity in hundreds of harbors. The thought that all this information, collected in the course of a lifetime, could be destroyed in an hour or so by fire terrifies Clapp. Friends are already at work trying to remedy this; they are raising $15,000 to build a fireproof structure.

CHAPTER XX

ATOM AGE

THERE can be no doubt of the fact that research men have moved us to the threshold of a new world; a world almost fantastically different from anything we now know. It will undoubtedly be recorded that a new era was ushered in with an explosion, an explosion of a very odd sort. No one heard it. No one saw it. Although it released 200,000,000 volts and ranked as the greatest man-made explosion in history, it still lacked power to tickle a mosquito.

It was the explosion of an atom.

The fact that it had occurred was revealed only by a photo plate.

To most readers such an explosion may appear to be as remotely important as a hailstorm on Mars. Yet this one is filled with alluring possibilities. Within a decade it may profoundly touch all of our lives. It may mean radical new airplanes and automobiles that run without fuel; furnaces that produce heat without coal or oil; ships that cruise endlessly with empty bunkers.

This accidental explosion has already touched off one of history's most dramatic races—a little-heralded competition for new knowledge among the earth's scientific great. Adolf Hitler took time out to set the staff of Berlin's Kaiser Wilhelm Institute on the job of investigating this atom that exploded so miraculously. To historians a hundred years hence that order may hold far more significance than the battle plans which swept his armies into a dozen countries.

Similarly, in Paris, Irene Curie and her husband, Frederick Joliot, got on the job.

In America no orders from a dictator were needed. Companies like General Electric, various universities and private laboratories appreciated the implications of that atomic explosion and joined the race. The stakes are great beyond the imagination: power in undreamed-of quantities.

But to mention these things here is to get ahead of our story, which begins 36 years ago when a bushy-haired little German-Swiss physicist challenged human thought with a daring concept. Matter and energy, said Albert Einstein, were very much the same thing. If the cohesive binding force that held together atoms in a pound of matter was suddenly set free, incredible amounts of power would be liberated. Dr. Einstein made calculations that indicated a pound of matter was the potential producer of *ten billion* kilowatt-hours of electricity! Thus, according to Einstein 12 pounds of totally destroyed matter would produce all electrical power consumed annually by the United States.

Enthusiastic science popularizers snatched at this fact and went happily to work figuring how many spoonfuls of water contained enough energy to drive a steamship across the Atlantic. Physicists smiled wryly. There was, they pointed out, one very great catch. A bombardment to smash this power out of a pound of atoms would require several times the ten billion kilowatt-hours of power that would be released. Atoms, they continued, were not packed tightly together. Therefore power-releasing hits would be rare. Einstein put the case aptly. Shooting at atoms, he said, was very much like shooting ducks on a dark night in the country where there weren't apt to be any ducks. There would be millions of misses for every hit. Hope of squeezing power from the atom appeared about as likely as the invention of a perpetual-motion machine. Then . . .

Dr. Otto Hahn, a worker at Berlin's Kaiser Wilhelm Institute, was bombarding uranium, a heavy metallic element, with neutrons—minute, electrically neutral fragments of matter. Atom smashing primarily consists of hurling tiny bits of matter at larger chunks of matter—atoms. The projectiles are shot forward by high voltages and when a direct hit is scored the atom flies apart, releasing its binding energy.

Hahn was working at this relatively routine business. Examining photo plates afterward the 60-year-old radiologist discovered that he had made a direct hit on a heavy, well-armored uranium atom and had split it in two. But the most significant thing: low-energy bullets had released 200,000,000 volts!

Appreciate the meaning of this: using small energies, Dr. Hahn had smashed into an atom, producing a tremendous amount of power. He had taken out far more energy from the uranium atom than he had put in! Perhaps atomic power wasn't such an idle dream after all.

When Hahn reported his epochal results, other physicists went excitedly about checking his claims. Workers at Washington's Carnegie Institution, Columbia University, Johns Hopkins and elsewhere sent neutrons slithering toward minute chunks of uranium—and they also saw 200,000,000-volt flashes on their photo plates.

There was one puzzling aspect about all this. If one atom released such vast amounts of power, why didn't some of this power go to smash a second, and a third atom? In other words, why wasn't there a chain action and a continuous flow of energy? Scores of scientists pursued this exciting train of thought. One of them was Niels Bohr, Danish Nobel Prize winner, who was working at the Institute for Advanced Study, at Princeton, New Jersey.

Bohr soon came forward with a suggestion. He pointed out that uranium as extracted from natural ore contains not only ordinary uranium, but two slightly altered forms, or isotopes, of uranium. Now, these two isotopes are important. An atom of ordinary uranium, heaviest of all elements, is built like a model solar system. Ninety-two electrons revolve about the dense nucleus. This nucleus contains 92 positively charged protons to balance the 92 negatively charged electrons. The nucleus also contains 146 neutrons. The atomic weight of ordinary uranium is 238. The two uranium isotopes are constructed in precisely the same manner, but one contains three fewer neutrons than the parent stuff, and the second has four fewer. Chemically and physically U-235 and U-234 are identical with more common U-238. (U is the chemical symbol of uranium.)

It was U-235, thought Bohr, that was exploding with such huge outbursts of energy. He also took note of the fact that a *slow*-moving neutron caused the explosion, whereas, a fast-moving one had no effect. One writer explained this admirably by comparing the situation to a golf game. A slow-moving ball frequently drops gently into the cup, but a fast-moving one hops over it. So with the neutron. According to Bohr the slow neutron dropped into the atom, which caused instability and resulted in an explosion. Too bad, said Bohr, that some of this U-235 wasn't available in pure form so the hypothesis could be tested.

His wish brought immediate action. Search for a means of extracting pure U-235 began at several places. Interest was whetted to razor edge by the stakes involved.

Two groups led the pack of searchers. One was headed by Dr. Alfred O. Nier, of the University of Minnesota. The other included Dr. H. C. Pollock and Dr. Kenneth H. Kingdon, of the Schenectady research laboratories of General Electric. Both groups used the same procedure in their work.

First they heated uranium in an electric furnace until it turned into vapor. Then they electrified this vapor and shot it through a magnetic field. The atoms, having different weights, were dragged down onto a platinum plate at different distances. Minute quantities of pure U-235 resulted.

A history-making moment was at hand. Both samples went to Columbia University for testing. Bombardment of the U-235 with slow neutrons began. Recording instruments told a vivid story of the high drama taking place within the bombardment chamber. A device for checking the explosions rattled like a machine gun. Another instrument that measured voltages resulting from the explosions moved to the 200,000,-000-volt mark and stayed there. As Bohr had assumed, explosions occurred in chain fashion, one atom giving up power to shatter a second, a second a third, etc. An all-important step toward atomic power had been achieved.

Calculations indicated the incredible amounts of power wrapped up in the silvery metallic element U-235. One pound, it developed, produced energy equal to that produced by 5,000,000 pounds of coal!

Further calculations showed an amazing thing. This power could be captured rather simply. No gigantic atom-smashing machine would be needed—not even to start the series of explosions. The highly unstable atoms of U-235 are constantly distintegrating and shooting off their own projectiles in the form of neutrons. All that was needed was a way to slow up these neutrons and permit them to find their target. And this trick could be accomplished merely by submerging some U-235 in ordinary water. The water would put a brake on the speed of the neutrons: permit them to hit the bull's-eye and start in motion the chain series of explosions. The water, meanwhile, would take up the heat produced by this violent action and change to steam. All that was needed for continuous power production was a constant supply of cool water. Cut off the water supply and the process would cease.

Power possibilities of this element are difficult to comprehend. An average house with a furnace that burns ten tons of coal per winter could get all the heat necessary for a 30-year period from a two-ounce piece of U-235. A similarly small piece might be sealed into the power plant of an automobile to provide energy as long as the car lasted. A two-pound piece would drive a submarine, and five pounds would propel an ocean liner.

Successful application of the power within this uranium isotope will almost surely necessitate redesigning of every navy in the world. Space and weight now devoted to fuel supplies will be given to heavier armor and more guns. Naval fueling stations, hitherto a necessity for any nation with pretensions to empire, will no longer be necessary. Fleets will have unlimited range.

At the moment, many things stand in the way of realization of such dreams. The basic scientific job has been done. Engineering work must follow. Uranium is synonymous with power. But how is the isotope to be extracted commercially from ore? And how, once extracted, is it to be utilized? Both questions pose large problems.

Uranium ore is plentiful in the world. There are large deposits in Canada, Colorado, the Belgian Congo, Germany, and elsewhere. U-235 is present in the ratio of one part for every 139 parts of common uranium. Getting this isotope out of the parent ore by the experimental methods employed at General Electric and at Minnesota is utterly out of the question. The cost would be staggering, and it would take an estimated 75,-000 years to collect a single pound!

Such obstacles will not, however, deter the search for cheaper extraction methods. Already an army of men is at work on this job. The United States Navy, General Electric and a dozen other research groups are working on it. Even though only a short time has elapsed since the inauguration of this effort, it is beginning to give results. From Stockholm, Professor Wilhelm Krasny-Ergen, worker at the Wenner-Grens Institute, reports that he has speeded up production 10,000 times by using a thermal diffusion tube. This improvement puts U-235 as a power producer just barely outside the limits of feasibility.

Investigators in this country are looking to the possibilities of the centrifuge. This machine sorts atoms as to weight by whirling them at high speeds, just as a cream separator whirls milk into component parts.

Most scientists feel that efforts in various directions will end successfully within a decade. But the technique for utilizing this amazing material also offers problems. The explosion rate of atoms must be carefully governed. Since it is possible that a few pounds of absolutely pure U-235 would go off with an earth-shaking explosion, impure alloys have been suggested. Ordinary uranium acts as a brake on the explosive process; cadmium is another possibility.

Solution of all the problems that attend this exciting new material may seem remote. And practical advantages from their solution may appear doubtful—as doubtful, in fact, as his pioneer electrical work must have seemed to Michael Faraday. But the point is that the barrier which once seemed insuperable has been broken. Atoms have given up enormous amounts of power. The task now is to collect enough of these atoms and find a way to harness their energy.

The day of atomic power, long awaited, has dawned.

While this wilderness is being explored, another group of men is busy in an equally bizarre field; the world that exists beyond our senses. It is a world filled with sights which our eyes can't see, smells which our noses can't detect, and sounds which our ears can't hear. It is a fascinating place denied to us because of the sharp limits of our perceptions.

We know audible sounds are put to a thousand purposes. We go to work to the blast of a factory whistle, communicate our thoughts with spoken words, and thrill to a stirring symphony. But can't *unheard* sounds, above and below the range of our ears, also work for us? The research man thinks so. Aren't there jobs for color bands invisible to the eye? Certainly, says the scientific investigator. Let's step into this forbidden territory.

Let's try and tune our ears to the sounds above and below the audible range. There is a vast world of sound here; a world of sounds too low for us to hear, yet heard by the fishes; of sounds too high for any but insect ears. We don't hear the miraculous cries of bats which guide them through dark caverns. They emit these cries 60 times a second. Sound waves that bounce back from obstacles serve to guide them. Thus a blindfolded bat flies perfectly; but one with plugged ears crashes frequently.

The average human ear can hear sounds that range from 16 cycles per second up to about 20,000. The lowest note on a large pipe organ stands at 16; the cry of a newborn infant 435; the highest note on a piano 4,700; the peep of a piccolo 4,572; the jangling of keys or the squeak of a door 16,000. At this point super sonics begin and go on to 40,000 cycles per second. Where super sonics leave off, ultra sonics begin.

An enormous amount of study has been devoted to the crashes, bangs and squeaks of this world—all unheard by our ears. Machines are on hand which convert inaudible to audible sound; and which make photographic records of frequencies too high to be heard. As is usually the case pure research was the forerunner of practical results.

Exciting applications have already been made and more exciting ones are on the way. The fathometer is an example of things now on hand. Sounds just on the fringe of audibility are shot downward from a ship, strike the bottom of the ocean and bounce back. The time elapsed is a measure of the depth, a detector of any hidden shoals.

The United States Navy has experimented extensively with ship-to-ship communications systems by means of super sonic sounds shot through the water; also with super sonic submarine detectors.

There is even a super sonic dog whistle. It is pitched too high to be heard by human ears, but not too high for the more sensitive ears of a dog. In this connection it should be noted that dogs hear many sounds inaudible to humans. This accounts for their suddenly becoming attentive when people in the same room have heard nothing. Possibly the dog has heard the high-pitched squeak of a mouse; the song of an unnoticed insect.

Machines are just now on the market which generate ultra sonic sounds of various frequencies. Before we attempt to understand the possible uses of such machines, let's glance for a moment at something which has been observed by everyone. Occasionally a deep note that issues from the radio speaker will set a strand of picture wire, or a metal ash tray vibrating. The ultra sonic generators do very much the same thing, but on quite a different scale.

They are used to agitate chemical solutions, thereby generating huge internal pressures. As a result of this super stirring many reactions are hastened. This feature appears to hold particular promise in the plastics industry. In some instances this unseen agitation caused by unheard sounds can shake molecules apart! When potassium permanganate is subjected to this violence it breaks up to form two new chemical compounds.

Experimentally, these super sonic sounds have been used to shake out gases dissolved in liquids. This is particularly important to makers of fine alloy steels—where a hidden air bubble can cause a failure. Researchers have also been able to destroy bacteria and red blood cells; and have—experimentally, at least—produced temporary sterility in the female.

A number of investigators are busy looking for potential uses of ultra sonics as a defensive weapon in warfare. A group of Chicago workers felt that these waves might be used to explode mines. All one needed was a wave to match the resonance point of the mine's detonator. They tried their hunch with a small mine placed in a swimming pool. An ultra sonic generator, placed 135 feet away, successfully set it off! Similar investigations are being carried on in the hope that the waves might be used to explode torpedoes.

Thus, research is getting under way in a noisy world mercifully denied our ears. What of the sights denied our eyes?

Look, for example, at the infra-red rays that lie just outside the visible spectrum.

These are the heating rays of the sun that come to us through 93,000,000 miles of space. With red-sensitive plates, photographers have been able to get pictures of heated flatirons in completely dark rooms. Military photographers have illuminated countrysides with "black light" and taken pictures on the darkest nights.

The infra-red rays produce heat which is particularly penetrating. Mightn't this feature have commercial applications? Westinghouse engineers asked themselves this question. Then they proceeded to build an electric lamp to generate infra-red light.

It was a superb new toy with which they performed a hundred entertaining stunts. They popped corn, baked eggs and cooked a steak in eight minutes with this invisible light! Then came serious business. Surely industry could find uses for this new magic. And it did.

A paint company noted that floor varnish would dry in 67 minutes instead of 24 hours when applied under a battery of these lamps. A building superintendent had a problem. He had 4,500 office doors that needed frequent refinishing. He found that infra-red would dry paint in twelve minutes instead of sixteen hours. The most dramatic application came in a Detroit auto factory. A motor manufacturer installed 10,000 of these lamps in a huge tunnel. Freshly painted car bodies pass through this cavern on a conveyor. They come out the other end dry—in a sixth the usual time.

The new light is being used to dry photographic negatives and prints; glues and inks. It isn't likely that infra-red lamps will ever displace the cook stove, but they should find uses in the home. Drying of laundry is one of the most obvious applications.

Let's swing to the other end of the spectrum: to the ultraviolet. Here, also, is light invisible to our eyes; but light which performs a thousand useful functions. In a sense ultra-violet is a "death ray"—but a death ray which kills microbes, not men. The exact mechanics by which this invisible light jars life out of bacteria is not known. But it does the job quickly and thoroughly.

Witness the magic it performs under a microscope. The action is projected onto a movie screen. The actors are paramecia—minute, slipper-shaped organisms which high-school biology students fish from stagnant ponds. As the scene opens the paramecia dart swiftly back and forth. Their speed increases. Then blisters appear on their bodies! Suddenly they explode!

Why? Because a beam of ultra-violet light was played upon them. Ultra-violet lamps strung over operating tables have materially reduced the number of infections that follow surgery. In hospital nurseries they sterilize the air; thereby preventing the spread of air-borne diseases. They are even being used in air-conditioning systems and home refrigerators. They are hastening the curing of meats and radically cutting the spoilage of bakery products caused by floating spores.

These two bands of light, at each end of the visible spectrum are but two of the miraculous sights hidden from our eyes. There are other things which we cannot see—but which are visible to newly built machines. Take the apparatus built by General Electric engineers which can *see* invisible gases. Poured from an apparently empty beaker, these gases show up on a screen as dark liquids!

The principle involved has many important applications. Leakage of mercury vapor from a huge turbine might be a costly item to a power company. A large installation may utilize a quarter of a million dollars' worth of mercury. Hundreds of dollars' worth of this valuable vapor can escape, undetected by the eye, unsmelled by the nose. But the new apparatus can spot the leak instantaneously.

It can also sniff out deadly carbon monoxide in a mine, or

in a vehicular tunnel.

General Electric's spectrophotometer is an astonishing instrument. It detects minute color differences which would baffle the eye of the most accomplished artist. To what purpose? Ordinarily these tiny color variations make little difference; but they are important to makers of colors, dyes, paints. The instrument was also used to match red inks with blood samples—thereby providing doctors with a convenient color scale used to spot anemia.

The photo-electric cell is another all-seeing marvel. One researcher gave a clue to its sensitivity. If the man in the moon were to light a match, he said, a photo cell could detect it. An exaggeration, perhaps, yet there is no denying the almost unbelievable sensitivity of these cells. We all know of the jobs they do better than men: leveling elevators, opening doors, sorting and counting packaged goods.

But what of the things they can do which men can't do? What of the sights they see, invisible to us? Look at one job recently assigned the photo cell. In a high-speed weaving mill, cloth flashes by a given point at the rate of ten thousand threads per second. To the human eye the threads are a blur. Yet if they get out of alignment a costly shutdown follows. It may be necessary to scrap hundreds of yards of material. Photo cells are eliminating this wastage.

Hooked on both sides of the weaving machine, they actually count two million threads every three minutes! If one cell counts more than its companion, the machine is brought into automatic alignment.

Placed inside a chimney, these cells can see when improper stoking is sending too much smoke into the air. Automatically, they open an air blast at the bottom of the furnace.

We all know how the X-ray can peer into the innards of little Willy and locate the safety pin he has swallowed; and how its shadows reveal the intimate details of a fracture. But do we know of the breath-taking advances made in recent months?

A new X-ray machine now in production takes pictures in a millionth of a second! See the significance of this. It can get a perfectly defined picture of a bullet as it crashes through a block of wood; or see what happens inside a golf ball at the moment of a club's impact. It can even see the internal parts of a gasoline engine going at top speed. Already research men are at work on an X-ray movie which will give a continuous record.

As things now stand scientists barely have a foot in the doorway leading to this world beyond our senses. From this unknown they have brought back scores of things to make life better and more pleasant in the world familiar to our eyes, ears, and noses. Tomorrow's explorations may completely revolutionize our way of life.

CHAPTER XXI

AGRICULTURAL RESEARCH

Last century Thomas Richard Malthus, British economist,
predicted that people of the earth ultimately faced starvation.
Population was increasing more rapidly than the capacity of
the soil to produce. By now, according to his calculations, we
should be dying off in large numbers. His theory looked
sound, but it omitted considering that very able person: the
agricultural researcher. Chemists and soil scientists have made
an acre of ground produce four times as much wheat as it did
in Malthus's day. Research men have produced hybrid corn,
bred cows and pigs to desired specifications and generally seen
to it that we have too much, rather than too little food.

Before we look at a few pieces of selected work in this field,
let's first examine that fabulous and omnipresent material:
soil.

There is a widespread tendency to look upon soil as a tem-
peramental, more or less unpredictable material. When it behaves properly farmers ride in expensive motor cars. When it
behaves badly there is a farm problem. This is superficial
thinking. The soil is astonishingly consistent, a living substance which, like men, passes through periods of youth, ma-
turity and old age. The soil nurses one civilization into full
flower while destroying another. It is the basis for all culture;
a substance which has astonishing influence on all our lives.

Is it accident that New England sends conservative men to
Congress? Is this an expression of the thrift and hard work as-
sociated with this section of the country? By no means, say soil
scientists. New England—and most all of the northeastern
United States—sits on the Grey-Brown podzolic soils. These

soils produce an almost endless variety of vegetable and animal life. Self-sufficiency on the farm is possible. This leads to conservatism. The black soils of the middle tier of states are different. By and large they are suitable for only one crop: grain. Farmers in this area are dependent on others. They must cooperate to survive. This pushes them toward the political left. Similar soils on the Russian steppes put people there almost solidly behind the Russian Revolution.

Schoolboys are taught that the Mason-Dixon Line divides North from South. Soil scientists laugh at such notions. The true boundary, they say, is the line of demarcation between the podzolic soils of the North and the red-yellow soils of the South. Men fought with their soil and not according to an arbitrary survey line. West Virginia, with Northern soil, tore away from its parent state to remain in the Union. A finger of Grey-Brown soil dips deeply into Eastern Tennessee. In this region men wore blue uniforms. Missouri, with the soils of both sides, put troops into both armies.

Men transplanted from native to a foreign soil often have vague feelings of discomfort. They are subject to emotional upsets. When they move in large numbers these suppressed feelings often flare into open violence. Such a thing happened in the settling of our own west. It was a wild west before new generations became adjusted.

What are these soils which so profoundly influence the music, art, literature and architecture of the men who live upon them? Even the simple soil is a masterpiece of biological and chemical mixing and blending, an expression of the geologic and climatic history of the area where it is found.

The construction of the few inches of topsoil which we regard so casually may have required anywhere from ten minutes to ten million years. The great alluvial rivers, the Ganges, Nile and Mississippi, build soil rapidly; but the slower process is the more interesting.

The starting point of any soil is, of course, rock. Weathering of the rocks which made today's soils began millions of years before man—that promising sprout on the evolutionary tree—appeared. Rain dissolved carbon dioxide from the air to make carbonic acid. This helped dissolve rock. Winter ice, forming in crevices, pried other bits apart. Bacteria, spores and seeds were introduced into this rocky débris by birds or by the wind. Life began. The Chernozem soils of the plains—producers of nearly all the world's bread—were gradually blackened by the accumulated rot of grasses. The forested podzolic soils took on a characteristic brown, and oxidized iron reddened the soils of the South. Where there was too little rainfall to permit vegetation, the rock weathered into sand to form deserts. By such processes the earth was presented with 36 great soil groups; and over 10,000 individual soils.

To support life satisfactorily a soil must contain an almost incredible variety of elements: nickel, cobalt, iron, iodine, potassium, to mention but a few. If nature has thoughtlessly neglected to include one of these things, this oversight is apt to have dramatic consequences. Iodine is lacking in the soils of Switzerland, the Himalaya region, and certain states around our own Great Lakes. Goitre is a pressing problem because the all-important thyroid gland in the neck requires iodine.

In one region in Australia cattle became wobbly kneed and died—despite the fact that they were pastured in belly-high clover. Cobalt was missing from the soil. It was necessary to cattle but not to clover. When fields were fed a small amount of this element they made safe grazing grounds. A similar cattle disease—"neck ail"—is encountered in Southeastern Massachusetts. This one has yet to be solved but it appears to trace to a deficiency of iron.

Exhaustion of these minerals presents a problem which cannot be lightly dismissed. All life depends on them. Prior to the advent of railroads and other means of transportation soils were reasonably constant. Whatever was removed was eventually replaced—in the form of vegetable and animal wastes.

Modern transportation allowed farmers to ship fertility away. What effect this may eventually have on human nutrition may only be guessed at. Some recent tests make significant suggestions.

Most people assume that an average amount of vegetables in diet will supply all essential minerals. Not necessarily. New research indicates that a head of cabbage grown on one soil may contain four times as much calcium as a similar head grown on another soil. One gathering of spinach may contain 30 times as much iron as another; and one carrot may contain 1,000 times as much iodine as a second.

Knowledge on this subject is, as yet, woefully lacking. A large-scale study jointly financed by New York State and the Federal government is just beginning at Cornell University.

Does man always destroy the land upon which he lives? One school of theorists holds this to be true. They point to the deserts of the Mediterranean area, the Near East and parts of China to support their thesis. Bad farming mined the soil of mineral elements until it could no longer produce crops. Then the civilization which it supported perished.

Another school refuses to accept this reasoning. Instead of land dragging down governments, they hold the reverse to be true. Corruption at the top, they say, led to high taxes. In an effort to survive farmers pushed land beyond its ability to produce. Fertility declined. In time the land refused to produce at all. Such a process, they hold, led to the fall of Rome and Greece.

At the same time there are examples of man improving the soil. Some areas of China have been farmed for thousands of years and are still highly productive. Crop yields on some soils in Puerto Rico are far higher now than they were 300 years ago. The dairy region of Wisconsin and the farm lands of central Pennsylvania are richer than they were when pioneers first pushed plows into the ground.

Every soil presents its own problems. The idea that a single fertilizer can cure all ills is as preposterous as assuming that a bottle of patent medicine cures all the ills listed on the label. Yet certain broad generalizations can be made. By and large soils of the Atlantic Seaboard are deficient in phosphorus; and the others are low in nitrogen.

At no spot in the United States has bad farming taken the toll that it has taken in the South. Over a century and a half cotton sapped the soil of fertility. It provided world trade dollars to build an industrial east and to liquidate a devastatingly expensive Civil War. But the one-crop system exacted a terrible price from the soil. Belatedly, this is being corrected. This unpublicized achievement ranks as one of the greatest— possibly *the* greatest—achievement of the New Deal.

The project is largely the work of Dr. Harcourt Alexander Morgan, tall, personable board chairman of the Tennessee Valley Authority.

Dr. Morgan drew up a soil balance sheet. The three basic essentials to all plant growth were potash, nitrogen and phosphorus. Potash represented no particular problem as it was generally prevalent in valley soils. Nitrogen could be captured from the air by legumes—plants such as red clover and lespedeza whose roots house nitrogen "fixing" bacteria. But these plants couldn't capture nitrogen unless phosphorus were present. Dr. Morgan collected some figures. In the course of a single year one pound of phosphate fertilizer properly used on plants would capture four pounds of nitrogen from the air!

And without phosphorus? There could be no life, either vegetable or animal. When it was lacking in the food of cattle their bones grew rubbery. They chewed at stray bits of wood. Eventually they died. Human beings who lacked this vital substance got rickets. The small stature of the Japanese and the widespread sterility encountered among women in India was credited to lack of phosphorus in the soil that provides them food. Japanese children born in California were almost invariably larger than their parents.

Figures indicate that at the present rate of depletion phosphorus will be completely exhausted from U.S. farm lands in 240 years, a brief period in terms of national history. Fortunately the country has adequate reserves of phosphate rock— a third of the world's known supply—from which replacements may be made.

Working second-grade phosphate deposits in Tennessee— the best rock had been exported to Germany prior to 1914— the TVA program got under way. Great electric furnaces at Muscle Shoals went into operation producing a highly concentrated phosphate fertilizer.

TVA's program was quietly introduced into the thinking of farmers, through the medium of county agricultural agents. Plant trees on steep slopes, ran the talk, and grass on the gentle slopes. Then phosphate and lime the bottom lands. Higher yields from the bottom lands would more than take care of any losses incurred by taking hillsides out of cultivation. And hillsides covered with grass wouldn't wash away. In addition to these benefits farmers would have new pastures for sheep and cattle which would help edge them away from the devastating corn-cotton economy.

Convincing results began to pile up as limited amounts of TVA phosphate went out to farmers in twenty states. Phosphated pasture accounted for a 146 per cent increase in milk production in one Minnesota test. In Virginia grass yields were increased 35 per cent—and pastures produced 77 pounds more beef per acre. But the most satisfying figures came in the Tennessee River area. Let Wheat Community tell the story of a thousand isolated communities where soil is on the way back.

Wheat Community is in the poor belt of Eastern Tennessee. There are 135 farms with a total of 12,000 acres. Prior to 1935 —when the program began—there were no telephones, electricity or hard roads. Hillsides had been corroded with rain, and "scalded knolls"—barren patches of clay hardpan—were general. Average farm income stood at $200 per year.

Phosphorus put new life into the soil. Altogether, acreage in soil-debilitating corn has been reduced 40 per cent. The number of cattle has increased 50 per cent. There are nine new pure-bred bulls to improve stock. Sheep are up 600 per cent, and hogs up 150 per cent. Land which would not grow red clover before phosphate came is now growing 86 acres of this valuable nitrogen-producing legume. Seven new houses have been built and five have been remodeled.

With about two-thirds of the farmers now in on the TVA program, there is enthusiasm and energy characteristic of a new country. Three years ago the community inaugurated a county fair, farmers contributing their services to build a large barn to display stock. An abandoned school was taken over for community activities. Wheat even had a pageant. Its title: Soil Builders.

A Ten-Year Plan drawn up by Community trustees indicates the kind of thinking now taking place. It doesn't envision a radio in every home and a car for every family. Thoughts are for the land which has won back the affections of the men who live on it. As goals for 1950 the plan calls for 3,000 acres to be terraced to prevent erosion. It wants 7,000 acres limed and phosphated; and 2,300 acres in permanent pasture.

Admittedly Wheat Community is an isolated example; yet it does indicate the kind of thinking going on in rural communities everywhere. The soil, so long neglected, is now getting the intelligent consideration that it demands.

This job is, to a large extent, one of education: a job of disseminating facts already assembled by researchers. Meanwhile, new facts are being assembled. The research men are busy devising better plant life, better farm animals, better methods of insect protection. Among these men no group is more fascinating than the plant breeders. See something of their problem.

You can't send a carrot to the hospital, and you can't vaccinate a field of beans. Yet these crops—and all plants for that matter—are as subject to disease as a delicate baby.

Cabbages have hernias, apple trees have tumors and cucumbers cankers. Insects spread virus diseases from one plant to another as mosquitoes spread malaria among men. Spores lie waiting in fields to attack crops as soon as they sprout; and fungus diseases are capable of destroying vegetables worth thousands of dollars in a single night's time.

For study of such problems the U.S. Department of Agriculture has recently completed a large research laboratory that occupies much the same position in the vegetable world that the Rockefeller Institute holds in the field of medical research. The laboratory—first of its kind in the world—is situated a few miles out of Charleston, South Carolina. Its job is to produce disease-resisting varieties of vegetables.

Vegetables, understand, don't just happen. They are designed as carefully as streamlined automobiles and electric egg beaters. Genes—minute factors of inheritance that go to make up the chromosome—are borrowed everywhere. Perhaps a bean from Bolivia is markedly resistant to a certain disease. Fine. Borrow the gene that determines this resistance and breed it into the line. Another gene will determine color, and a third taste. String them together in a necklace pattern and you have a new chromosome—and a new bean.

Plant breeders are an exciting crew. Like politicians, they hold out the alluring promise of a more abundant life. The only difference is that the plant breeders are delivering. As a nation we are eating better food than we did a generation ago. Thank the plant breeder. Largely due to his efforts in suppressing vegetable diseases, we now have an enormous variety of year-round foods.

Look at some striking figures: In the past two decades acreage planted to the commercial asparagus crop has risen 400 per cent. Lettuce is up 500 per cent; carrots and spinach are up 600 per cent; beets and peas up 1,000 per cent.

To find the disease-resistant characteristics required, plant explorers tramp the out-of-the-way places of the world. You'll find them pawing through the vegetable stalls in Bagdad and on the scraggly hillside farms in Afghanistan; under the hot sun of Persia and on the slopes of the Andes. They are not looking for finished products in vegetables. They are satisfied if they can find a single wanted characteristic. Beans from Turkey may taste like laces from high-top boots, but if they are immune to a certain disease the plant explorer cherishes them. Good eating qualities can be bred in later.

An example will illustrate how they work: The cantaloupe crops of the irrigated regions in the Southwest were being destroyed by powdery mildew. Thousands of acres of melons had been ruined and the disease epidemic appeared to be barely getting under way. Bankruptcy faced the whole farm population.

The late Dr. Ivan Jagger of the U.S. Department of Agriculture was assigned to the job. His jumping-off place was a scrubby little melon that he found in India. It was small, tasteless and subject to rot. From a market man's point of view it was utterly valueless. But to Jagger it had one brilliant feature: powdery mildew didn't touch it. He crossed this unpromising import with good domestic varieties; and back-crossed the resulting progeny with the parents. For four years this went on, but finally the desired product emerged: a sweet, disease-resistant melon. Like a hero in an old-fashioned melodrama, he completed the job in time to lift mortgages on a thousand homes.

Similar pieces of work have been done for the lettuce growers. The Louisiana sugar-cane crop was saved from a mosaic disease, caused by a virus, the same type of organism that causes yellow fever and infantile paralysis in human beings.

Work at Charleston began after the Bankhead-Jones Act made $135,000 available for the purchase of a 435-acre farm and construction of laboratories. Thirteen Southern states co-operated in the project. In the spring of 1936 these states sent representatives to Charleston to lay out work.

One man suggested cotton research. Enough work being done elsewhere with this crop, the delegates decided. Another suggested sugar cane. The same thing obtained here. Gradually discussion turned to vegetables. The South had never been a vegetable-growing country. People subsisted on a diet of sweet potatoes, collards, rice and cowpeas. Share-croppers grew cotton to their doorsteps, then bought food, woefully lacking in necessary minerals and vitamins, at plantation commissaries.

The reason the South didn't grow vegetables, delegates knew, was because of the vast array of plant diseases ready to pounce on any crop planted. Winters aren't severe enough to kill organisms left in the ground from year to year. If these diseases could be whipped the South might be plowed into a gigantic new truck garden for the nation. New crops would attract new industries—principally canning. And a better diet would be provided for the home folks.

These arguments were winning. Vegetables it would be, said the delegates. By vote they selected specific problems, and decided the laboratory should devote its time and attention to tomatoes, cabbage, beans, watermelons, peas and sweet corn. Bacteriologists, pathologists and chemists would study the specific diseases that attacked these crops, and botanists and geneticists would see what they could do about breeding resistant strains. Dr. Bryan L. Wade, bushy-haired young West Virginian, took charge. He had bred hardy peas in Mexico for commercial seed companies and had worked all over the United States for the Department of Agriculture.

Understand a little about crossing plants, before we get along to individual research problems. In producing hybrid corn, tassels (the male organs) and silks (female) must be protected to prevent haphazard fertilizations. A paper bag clamped over the tassel and a glassine envelope over the silk gives this protection. When one stalk is to be crossed with another, pollen is shaken from the tassel and dusted over the silk of the second. With beans the problem is slightly different. The bud, which contains both male and female parts, is opened with tweezers. Next it is castrated—by removal of stamens. Pollen taken from another plant is dropped into the bud, which is then sealed with a glassine bag.

One of the first jobs undertaken at Charleston was production of a completely new watermelon. The watermelon needed redesigning. It was too big. The usual melon shipped by the South weighed 40 pounds—too bulky to fit in the refrigerator of the average family. Furthermore, the commercial watermelon needed more sugar. These were consumer problems. Producer problems were even larger.

There are a number of diseases that prey on the South's watermelon belt—which produces over 30 million melons a year—but Fusarium wilt is the biggest problem. This fungus disease is carried by seeds. Surface water spreads the fungi from one field to another, and melon patches are known to have been contaminated by mud carried on shoes. The fungus survives in the soil as long as twenty years.

Wilt is a quick worker. It stops the circulatory system of the plant and whole fields die overnight. In one Iowa area formerly devoted to watermelons, 90 per cent of the acreage has been abandoned. Florida growers partially escape ravages of the disease by planting only in virgin soil.

The first step in breeding the desired small, resistant melon was to get word out to plant explorers. Seeds began to arrive, particularly from old countries like China, Persia, and Africa, home of the watermelon. Plants that have survived a thousand or so years in such places have high disease resistance.

Turkey sent citrons, watermelon relatives, whose preserved rind is used in fruitcakes. They are almost immune to wilt diseases. Working outside in summer and in greenhouses in winter, the plant breeders made over 300 watermelon crosses. They have produced a small melon that survives in heavily contaminated soil. As it stands today it needs more sugar. This quality will be added and then the country should have a new dessert; a small, sweet melon not much larger than a good-sized honeydew—a tough customer that the farmer can plant without fear.

Corn is another problem in the South—as everyone knows who has eaten it south of the Mason-Dixon Line. Corn-ear-worms attack sweet corn to such an extent that farmers cannot plant this crop. So they plant field corn, gather it in the milk stage and pass out for human consumption a corn meant for horses. It is tough and tasteless—so tough and tasteless that not even the ear-worms will eat it.

The breeder's problem here is to get a corn that will have the ear-worm resistance of field corn and the sweetness of Northern eating corn.

A crop grown in a greenhouse patch is sweet and toothsome. Worms attack only the tips of the ears. It should be ready after about two more generations. Then the precious seeds—worth several times their weight in gold—will go into "in-crease plots." From these plots bushels of seeds will go out to state stations for further increase, and eventual distribu-tion to farmers.

One of the luckiest happenings in the history of the labora-tory came on Thanksgiving Day, two years ago. In a few hours' time thermometers plunged down 52 degrees to a point well below freezing, and stayed there for about a week. All vege-table crops in the neighborhood were frozen out. Dr. Wade went out to examine a four-acre field of peas that should have been destroyed too. Far the greater part of the crop was gone. But in the middle of the field a few score plants were upright, uninjured! Had the plant breeders accidentally hit upon a cross that would withstand severe frosts? It looked that way. Both parents of the cross were dead, so cold resistance ap-peared to be something new to the line.

This set the breeders off on a new tack. The idea of a cold-resistant pea had engaging possibilities. It meant that winter vegetable crops could be pushed farther north and that large new areas could be opened for planting. It also meant that instead of planting in the Mid-South on January first, plantings could be made several weeks earlier. This would get crops to market earlier, while prices were still high.

In order to be able to produce any temperatures wanted, Dr. Wade built a special refrigeration apparatus. Cooling coils are built into a box which is placed over the plants. The compressor is carried on a trailer. Thus, at any time of the year, artificial frosts can be produced to test hardiness of new strains. Seeds of this new stock have already gone out to state stations for additional testing. While this project doesn't necessarily promise February peas at July prices, such a thing is a distinct possibility.

Tomatoes, favorite crop of home gardeners, are getting a great deal of attention at the Charleston laboratory. Chief reason for this is that in the thirteen Southern states this crop is subject to a host of diseases—nailhead blight, root rot, mosaic disease and others. Shippers are handicapped by the fact that inroads of disease cut the harvest season to three weeks, whereas Northern and Western farmers enjoy a six-week harvest season. At the end of three weeks, diseases have so damaged plants that fruit is valueless in the market.

At the outset, plant explorers began sending tomato seeds from Afghanistan, India and elsewhere. A special expedition went out to South and Central America. Plants grown from seeds that came back produced fruit that only the trained eye would recognize as tomatoes. Some were pear-shaped; others grew fuzz; and still others were greenish little knots no larger than marbles. Some had white stripes, and others grew in clusters like grapes. But each one had some desirable characteristic.

The 12-acre tomato patch on the farm probably contains the greatest variety of tomatoes ever assembled on earth. Hundreds of crosses grow in this field. Some are inedible and some hold out no promise. They will be discarded. But one newcomer has great possibilities. Even in the most heavily contaminated fields it survives for four weeks. That extra week in the market will mean hundreds of thousands of dollars for shippers of early tomatoes. This tomato isn't yet ready for general distribution. More tinkering with its chromosomes will make it even more resistant before it is ready for our spring salads.

Every phase of vegetable breeding is being investigated at Charleston. In the bacteriological laboratory, workers are growing the various fungi, bacteria and viruses that raise havoc in the vegetable world. Cultures, artificially produced, are kept on hand to contaminate soil and test resistance of new crosses. An effort is being made to standardize exact doses of bacteria and fungi necessary to produce disease in plants. Armed with this information, plant breeders will have a measure of immunity—something like the Schick test, which offers a measuring stick for diphtheria immunity in children.

Greenhouses, models of efficiency, have elaborate temperature and humidity controls and are equipped with lights for growing plants at night. Soil sterilizers are used to kill off any unwanted organisms in the ground.

Even such a modest achievement as a cold-resistant cabbage would defray cost of the work many times over. If research at the laboratory can cut the enormous toll taken by disease in the vegetable world, that is tantamount to saying that farmers can produce more food while expending no greater amount of labor. This means lower prices. It means better diet for the South, and benefits to the nation as a whole.

CHAPTER XXII

SAVE IT!

For the chemist the ideal world is a world where everything
is completely used up, a world with no slag piles, chimney
wastes, or refuse heaps. He lies awake nights trying to worry
out uses for things normally thrown away. Now he is getting
his big chance. He is starting a large-scale attack on the world's
largest pile of débris—the agricultural wastes produced by
American farms. In the pile there are, among other things, 85
million tons of various straws, and 100 million tons of corn
stalk and leaves. It contains 240,000 tons of peanut shells and
25,000 tons of walnut shells. If we include United States insular possessions, three million tons of bagasse—stalk left
after sugar has been pressed from cane—must be added to the
heap.

The farmer, to be sure, makes a few ineffectual pecks at this
mass of rubbish. He turns his pigs in fields and lets them "hog
down" fodder. He uses some cobs for kindling and burns
others to charcoal to supplement diet for his stock. Baled
straw—to be used for animal and human bedding—brings
him barely enough to pay for his trouble; and bagasse left
from his cane goes chiefly to fire boilers in sugar mills.

Such goings on make the chemist shudder. He looks on
these leavings as source material for brilliant new fabrics,
plastics and lacquers. He would convert them into motor
fuel, paper and valuable chemicals. For him, today's junk is
tomorrow's gold.

Until about 50 years ago cottonseeds were thrown into
rivers or allowed to rot in fields. Oil squeezed from them
today goes to make an annual $100,000,000 worth of soap,

oleomargarine and cooking fat. Over 100,000 tons of Louisiana bagasse go to feed that lusty baby—the new wallboard industry. In Hawaii they're using the same material to make artificial silk. There are 40 United States plants which convert thousands of tons of straw into grey chipboard—used to line egg crates and keep freshly laundered shirts from wrinkling. Carbon made from refuse nut shells is used for gas masks, and licorice root, from which flavoring has been extracted, is processed into building board. These things barely scratch the surface, though they do represent industry totaling millions of dollars. The chemist wants to sic his new magic on wastes and build industries worth billions.

If this idea has a prophet, that prophet is Dr. Orland R. Sweeney, head of the chemical engineering department at Iowa State College—agriculture's Harvard. Dr. Sweeney, 58, is white-haired, cherubic. With the enthusiasm of a cypress-swamp evangelist, he has been preaching utilization since early this century. Converted to the cause of conservation by Gifford Pinchot and Theodore Roosevelt, he went them one step better. Why not save other things besides trees, he asked. Agricultural wastes, for example?

Sweeney, then a youngster teaching chemistry at Ohio State, listed twenty wastes which he thought could be processed into a board suitable for partitions, insulation and plaster base. Strangest waste product: refuse removed from cow stomachs at packing houses. Proud of his little intellectual exercise, Sweeney marched into the office of the university president. He was cold-shouldered out with directions to come back when his ideas were past the talk stage.

Back in his laboratory, Sweeney puttered and stewed and finally produced a board made out of bagasse. His researches hadn't gotten beyond this when the first World War started and he was assigned to work on poison gases.

At the end of the war he took a job on the faculty of Iowa State and got down to work in earnest. Result of these early investigations was a chemical called furfural, derived from oat hulls and corncobs. This substance is used in the plastics industry and thousands of pounds are required to remove sludge from motor oil. Largely as a result of Sweeney's work one of the biggest breakfast foods manufacturers added a furfural-extracting plant to consume the mountains of oat hulls produced at its Cedar Rapids plant.

Sweeney next turned to a cornstalk building board. He shredded, boiled and pressed stalks and leaves until he had a board that satisfied him. Result here was a plant at Dubuque whose huge tonnage goes chiefly to one of the big mail order houses. After this success Sweeney decided he needed help. The refuse pile was too big for a one-man attack.

He told his story to his friend, Herbert Hoover, then Secretary of Commerce. Why couldn't the government participate in this business, he asked. Use up a lot of wastes, give the farmers more income, and bring industry to the corn belt. Little industries sprinkled through rural regions would help even out the bumps that came when farm prices slumped. Mr. Hoover was sympathetic. The idea appealed to his engineering mind. He got a $50,000 appropriation to be spent jointly by Iowa State College and the Bureau of Standards.

Benefits from this feeler expenditure were great enough for the Department of Agriculture to take over in 1931. In 1935, money was forthcoming for a compact little brick building, The Agricultural By-Products Research Laboratory, which was located on the campus at Ames.

Already the Ames chemists have developed a number of new products and are working on a host of others. Step into the work room of T. R. McElhinney to see how things go. Tom McElhinney is a lanky, jut-jawed Iowa farm boy who hails from Waterloo. He took chemistry at Iowa State, got a job in the laboratory when he graduated, and was assigned to work with plastics.

Trucks dumped assorted débris—corncobs, stalk, straw,

bagasse—in McElhinney's barn-like lab. He chopped them up and treated them in cookers with various chemicals. In powerful presses he'd put the resultant messes under pressures up to 3,500 pounds to the square inch. Like as not they would stick in molds and have to be removed with a cold chisel. Other times they'd be runny and gooey. Finally, he made a plastic out of bagasse that looked good. It was hard without being brittle, satisfactorily water-resistant, and had the lustre of a piece of highly polished marble.

The plastic was all right, but what about costs? McElhinney started out with one thing in his favor here. Bagasse, unlike most other farm wastes, offers no particular problem of collection. Cane is hauled to mills and refuse material from thousands of acres is automatically collected in one neat pile. To be well over on the conservative side he figured cost of bagasse at $8 a ton, whereas board mills are able to get all they can use at $4 to $5 a ton.

After toting up all material costs, the finished powder, which is pressed into various shapes, figured out at 5 cents a pound—half the price of the cheapest plastic on the market. Cheapness of the new material opens up vast new fields denied present plastics because of cost. It can be pressed into tiles for kitchens and bathrooms that are cheap enough to compete with better grades of lumber. Door frames, wall panels, baseboard and even roof tiles are other possibilities. Two of the three largest motor makers are already at work with the new material, testing its adaptability to single slab dashboards, steering wheels, etc.

Upstairs from the plastics lab Drs. G. H. Nelson, chemist, and Robert Straka, bacteriologist, are off on another project. At the outset they decided it would be nice if they could find bacteria, molds or fungi which would eat away unwanted materials in stalks and straws and leave pure cellulose for paper making. Following their microscopic hounds, they went far afield of the project originally outlined.

Lignin, which accounts for about 25 per cent of all pulpy vegetable matter, offered greatest difficulties. No microbes would touch it. Nelson, who hadn't the slightest idea about why they turned up noses at this food, started out on a long-range study of the substance. Very little is known of the chemistry of lignin beyond the fact that it appears to be the glue that binds cellulose together in trees, cornstalks, hollyhocks, and other vegetable matter.

Wanting to see how it reacted with various metals, he stirred pure lignin into a solution which contained some of the common salts of iron. When he filtered the solution, the filter paper was covered with a blackish substance! Lignin had precipitated about 98 per cent of the iron out of the solution.

Realize the rôle iron plays in water and you'll catch the meaning of this. Iron, which imparts an evil taste and color to water, is disastrous to textile, paper, ice and laundry industries. It discolors bath fixtures, clogs pipes, and is otherwise an expensive nuisance in municipal water systems. Next to the suppression of bacteria, it offers the biggest problem in the life of any water company.

Thousands of tons of the mineral zeolite, lime, soda ash, and other iron removers are used annually in the United States. From advance data so far available, lignin does the job more cheaply, and more efficiently.

This material can be extracted from corncobs, stalk and straw, is also available in paper-mill wastes. At present it has only three uses. Since it extracts moisture from the air it is utilized to a small extent to keep down dust on country roads. The plastics industry uses a little. A minute amount goes to make synthetic vanilla extract. This work opens up an enormous new outlet.

While Nelson was making this discovery Dr. Straka kept at the problem of fermentation. Scores of jars containing a grim-looking black mash made of cornstalks and other débris, bubbled away. When no cultures were found which wanted to eat lignin, Straka began to analyze gases given off by fermentation. Most of the bottles were giving off hydrogen, a small amount of carbon dioxide, and a large amount of methane—inflammable marsh gas. An idea struck. Why couldn't farmers use waste straw and cornstalks to manufacture their own fuel gas? Use it in their cook stoves and light their homes with it?

Straka weighed bottle charges of chopped stalk, and metered the gas produced. Resulting figures indicated that a ton of fodder would produce 10,000 cubic feet of gas. Since domestic consumers of manufactured gas pay an average of $1.31 a thousand for this fuel, Straka's fodder has an indicated gas value of $13.10 a ton.

For the average home, Straka figures that it would be necessary for the farmer to fork 50 pounds of fodder into the fermenter each day. The tank, which would be about eight feet in diameter and six feet deep, would require cleaning every four or five months. Scores of wrinkles have yet to be ironed out before such a system can be made completely fool proof. At the moment a satisfactory tank is giving trouble. Metals seem to inhibit bacterial action, so work now is progressing with tile and brick containers.

Straka is also thinking in terms of larger units to supply the gas requirements of small, farm-belt towns. Carbon dioxide produced by the fermentation could be compressed into dry ice, and residuary mash could be pressed into board. Then the chemist's ideal would be achieved. Nothing would be wasted.

Down the corridor from Straka's laboratory another man, Dr. Nandor Porges, is making microbes jump through hoops. He sets them to work on corn sugar, watches results. This sugar isn't, of course, an agricultural waste. Rather, it is an agricultural by-product. But new uses for corn sugar can be translated into more farm income, and more industry for towns and cities. That, after all, is the chief aim of the laboratory. Dr. Porges, smiling and rotund, has made his microbes perform astonishing tricks. Money-making tricks. Setting them to work under various conditions of pressure, vacuum and heat, he has produced a large array of new chemicals.

He has devised a radical new method for producing calcium gluconate—used in tanning, metallurgy, toothpaste, human and veterinary medicine. In medicine this chemical is used to quickly supply calcium which the body may need. The old rule of a tooth a baby need no longer hold. Although the material is getting clinical trials for a host of human ills, most of this work is still in an experimental stage. Best results to date have come in cow medicine. Due to the drain on body calcium imposed by calf bearing, cows frequently topple over dead after delivering their young. Calcium gluconate is assimilated so rapidly that a single shot will revive them in a few minutes. Until a few years ago this substance fetched $150 a pound. Now, since Porges has tamed microbes and put them to work, a small commercial plant in Missouri is producing the material for 50 cents a pound.

A similar project—again using microbes to do the work of men and machinery—had reduced the price of a chemical curiosity called sorbose from $450 a pound to $11 a pound. This is the parent substance from which Vitamin C (anti-scurvy) is derived.

The ideal of by-products chemists is to successfully make paper out of agricultural refuse. Reasons for this are obvious. The United States consumes over 12,000,000 tons of paper a year. If cellulose for this production were derived from farm wastes it would make a handsome hole in the waste pile.

There are numerous catches to achievement of this goal at the moment. For one thing paper making demands cheap power—something not available in the farm belt where the wastes are produced. For another, pulp prices in recent years have been so depressed that hardly any pulp mills could operate profitably. These twin factors have ruled out utilization of farm wastes only in so far as present paper-mill processes and methods are used. At Ames, chemists are seeking radical new methods of production. They know that they *can* make excellent paper out of nearly any of the wastes they work with. Hawaii has a mill operating on bagasse, and Italy and South American countries have subsidized mills using straw. So it is purely a question of price.

Paper gets the attention of more men in the Ames laboratory than any other problem. Their estimates show that within a ten-mile radius of almost any spot in the corn country enough stalk and leaf is available to support continuous activity in a 50-ton-a-day paper mill. They have made hundreds of strong and handsome papers but have yet to whip the bugaboo of price.

The research men at Ames have made punk for lighting firecrackers out of corncobs, and have even made a corncob incense which might be useful in perfuming air of theatres. They have subjected chicken feathers to destructive distillation, in the search for new drugs and chemicals, and have sought uses for nut shells and citrus refuse. They dream in terms of new industries scattered through rural regions, more dollars for the farmer, and a whole array of new building materials, textiles and plastics for the home.

This work at Ames gives an indication of the shape of things to come. Meanwhile, the farm belt has before it an excellent example of how research can be translated into new industry. Several years ago research men—notably Dr. Birdseye—began experimenting with processes for quick-freezing foods. In the end they produced a completely new method for food preservation. At first their findings were utilized solely by large food packers. Now it is proving its value to individual farmers.

These low-temperature plants are spreading everywhere. Farmers rent individual lockers. In summer when fruits and vegetables are going begging, farmers put them away, freeze them rock hard and eat them months later. Chickens, turkeys, hogs, cows and sheep are similarly treated.

This brand-new industry has grown with astonishing speed. Four years ago it was virtually nonexistent. No one—not even the new national association of locker owners—knows how many plants there are today.

A Department of Agriculture survey which covered 38 states, counted 1,861. This was two years ago. Since locker plants were being built at the rate of over fifty a month, the survey was out of date before it was even published. Good guessers say that there are probably 3,000 of them today, and that about a million families are participating in benefits.

Quick-frozen foods must not be confused with slow-frozen foods. Slow freezing is what happens to fruits and vegetables left on the vine after frost comes. Generally speaking, they turn black and get watery and tasteless, because slow freezing creates large ice crystals in individual cells. These crystals puncture cell walls and vital juices leak away. But when peas, beans and pork are frozen quickly by temperatures down to 30 or 40 degrees below zero, only minute crystals form and these leave cell walls intact. After being thus frozen, and stored at zero temperature, they keep perfectly fresh for months. Even the most exacting tastes are unable to distinguish between fresh and frozen foods.

No one is sure where this new business got started. Most people think that it originated on the Pacific Coast, and that it began when farmers started asking ice plants to let them rent space to store meat, eggs and poultry. As knowledge increased about handling quick-frozen foods, plants devoted solely to lockers began to spring up. Date the beginning of the industry with 1935 and you won't be far wrong.

As they stand today, the plants represent the first significant change in recent times in the handling and storage of farm foods. Benefits, of course, can be enormous. The farm wife escapes the drudgery of canning vegetables, preserving fruits and cold-packing meats. And the family escapes eating the products of her toil. Butchering of cows and hogs, once limited to the winter, can now take place at any time. The farmer has a new variety of foods to eat the year round, and most of these foods are far richer in vitamins than his usual diet.

Figures of savings that accrue to locker users vary widely. A retail butcher can put up a convincing story that there is no saving, and a locker-plant operator can busy his pencil to prove that the average family gets ahead at the rate of $100 per year. One unbiased survey indicated $30.

One of the really elegant plants will be fancied up with glazed tile, enameled lockers and comfortable waiting rooms. It will have a thousand or more food compartments, each leased by the year. To get some notion of how it operates, let's start with an individual farmer renting one of these lockers.

During the summer, when pork prices were low, he decided to butcher a hog and lay in a supply of reasonably priced meat for his family. By butchering then instead of waiting for the cold weather, he saved a large feed bill. Since he was busy with his crops he decided to turn the whole job over to the locker plant.

In his own truck, he delivered the hog. The butcher in attendance took charge. For a fee of $1 he slaughtered the animal and hung it in the "chill" room. Body heat was dissipated over the course of two or three days in this room where temperature is held at 34 degrees. Then the hog was hauled down and taken to the cutting room. An expert butcher cut the animal up. He ground scrap into sausage (and would even have stuffed it into casing if desired), rendered lard, sliced off chops, and so forth.

Chunks of meat were wrapped in waterproof paper, enough in each package to make a meal. Each was dated and labeled as to contents. All these were listed on an inventory card. For this service the farmer, of course, paid a price. It cost him 3 cents a pound to have his lard rendered; cutting and wrapping came to 1 cent a pound; sausage grinding another cent.

After wrapping, the packages were placed in a wire basket and taken to the sharp-freeze room. In this place a minus-30-degree temperature is maintained. A day or so here froze the meat solidly. Then packages were moved to the locker room, which is held at zero.

Vegetables require speedy, careful handling if garden freshness is to be preserved. This job usually falls to the housewife. Peas and asparagus will illustrate how it is done. Asparagus is gathered and carried to the kithen, where it is cleaned. Then it is immersed in boiling water for two minutes. This is a vastly important step. This scalding inhibits the action of ferments which cause spoilage. Next the asparagus is dried and packed in containers—perhaps one-quart waxed cartons. Peas are handled in much the same manner but packed in cheaper ice-cream buckets.

After packing, these vegetables are chilled in the home icebox until ready to be transported to the locker plant where they are placed in the sharp-freeze room for a few hours before being stored in the locker.

The lower the temperature maintained in the storage room, the better for the products. At 40 below zero the action of ferments ceases almost entirely, and vegetables and meats will keep indefinitely. But cost of maintaining such a temperature is far too high. Zero appears to be satisfactory from all points of view. At this level the action of ferments is only half what it is at 15 degrees F. Chemical action goes on but at too slow a pace to do much damage. Most foods will keep for six months to a year.

Some of the more complete locker plants have all the necessary equipment for the farm wife. She can bring her vegetables to the plant in baskets. A small fee permits her to use pea shellers, steam kettles, etc.

Although they were designed primarily for use by farmers, city and town people are renting about a quarter of the million lockers now in service. Since they don't raise their own food for storage they must buy it. Boarding-houses, hospitals, hotels and clubs are enthusiastic locker users. Vegetables are picked up in the summer when they are cheap. Meats are ordinarily purchased from the manager of the locker plant. He will buy a carload of beef at wholesale prices and resell it to his patrons—charging a brokerage fee of 1 or 2 cents a pound. Then the locker-plant butcher will cut it up to the purchaser's specifications.

Memphis, Toledo, Des Moines, Lancaster, Pennsylvania, and other cities already have such storage places, and they are springing up elsewhere. Urbanites apparently like the idea of having a cache of food.

In most instances the city plants offer a variety of services that aren't encountered in rural districts. Some of them maintain a delivery service—charging a cent a pound. Others retail a complete line of commercial quick-frozen products. This allows patrons a variety of foods beyond those held in their lockers.

Packers are generally friendly to the idea. Farmers have never been important buyers of meat and the idea of selling several hundred pounds of beef at a time to city people has its appeal.

These plants are frequently adjuncts to other businesses. Cold-storage warehouses or ice-cream plants, for example. Many Midwest creameries have added locker plants and offer dairy farmers the advantages of home deliveries. Trucks that gather milk from farms also deliver food from the farmer's locker. Even retail meat shops have added locker plants.

Other plants are privately owned, or owned by cooperatives. Costs of construction vary, but $10,000 to $12,000 is a fair price for a plant containing 300 or 400 lockers. Owners or operators of these plants generally charge $10 to $12 a year locker rental. Extra income is derived from the service charges already mentioned. Some plants pick up enough extra money to pay their power bills by storing fur coats during the summer.

Almost anything can be stored—even butter and eggs—provided certain simple rules are followed; and provided the locker renter has taken care to select varieties of vegetables that are well adapted to freezing. Broccoli, corn on the cob, spinach, Brussels sprouts are excellent. Peaches require quick handling to prevent their turning black but raspberries, blueberries and strawberries handle nicely.

Berries and fruits are usually packed in dry sugar or sugar syrup. This keeps oxygen away from the surface so that they don't blacken. In some cases patrons prefer to bake fruits into pies and then store the pies. Nearly all perishable foods can be handled in the locker plants, with the exception of tomatoes, pears and watermelons.

Greatest strides have been taken by the locker operators in the Midwest. The first plant in Iowa was built in the southwestern corner of the state at Creston, in 1934. Today there are over 400. Illinois built its first one in 1935 and today has well over a hundred. The South is still virgin territory and so is New England.

CHAPTER XXIII

PESTS

Few of us drop furtive tears when an epidemic strikes down a field of wheat; and no one goes into mourning for a crop of tomatoes destroyed by disease. The drama of sudden death in the vegetable world is lost on the average person. Yet plants do have an incredible variety of ailments; ailments that pick the pocket of the farmer, keep food from the mouths of the hungry and generally impose a crushing economic burden.

A disease as relatively unknown as leaf curl destroys 320,000 bushels of peaches, and halo blight takes 135,000 bushels of snap beans. Spot blotch removes 800,000 bushels of barley from the market, and stem rust will take 80,000,000 bushels of wheat. Added together, plant diseases and insect pests cost the nation three billion dollars a year!

Credit for the fact that things are no worse is due to the quarantine service maintained by the Department of Agriculture. In the vegetable world it performs jobs similar to those done for human beings by the United States Public Health Service. To keep plant equivalents of plague, typhus and cholera out of the country it maintains a number of counterparts of Ellis Island. All plants allowed to enter undergo rigid inspection, and some spend four years in quarantine stations as closely guarded as Alcatraz.

Reasons for these precautions are understandable when one beholds the depredations of an imported pest. The boll weevil, sent us by Mexico, destroys $120,000,000 worth of cotton a year. Sugar-cane mosaic slipped into the fields of Louisiana. It caused wholesale destruction, handing planters a bill for $100,000,000 in one six-year period. So the men who guard the country against such pests aren't dealing with petty annoyances.

Perhaps the lady who arrives in Miami on the plane from Cuba is inordinately annoyed by the inspector who takes her corsage of roses and tosses it into an incinerator. But that corsage might contain black flies that would go through Florida citrus orchards as speedily as fire through a pine woods. The importer who brings in a cargo of cheap baseballs from Japan is highly indignant when his bill of goods is barred. But the baseballs are stuffed with cotton-gin refuse, and the cotton seeds are contaminated with larvae of the pink bollworm. A pop fly knocked by a youngster into an Alabama cotton field might let these pests loose on the South. Were the bollworm let free to add his ravages to those of the boll weevil it is possible that the South would no longer be able to grow its greatest money crop.

To guard against entrance of these pests and a thousand others like them, the Department of Agriculture maintains fourteen stations on the Mexican border, six on the Canadian border and twenty-six at various Atlantic, Gulf and Pacific ports. Before this activity began in 1912, the United States was presented with a host of pests. A fly brought by Hessian troops during the Revolution accounts for a yearly $13,000,-000 damage to wheat. China sent us the chestnut blight. The gypsy moth, deliberately imported by a man interested in breeding it with the silkworm to produce a hardy strain, has done upwards of $20,000,000 damage since its arrival.

The quarantine service strives to prevent repetition of these costly tragedies. Elaborate precautions are taken with almost every ounce of vegetable matter that enters the United States. Cotton will illustrate. Millions of pounds of long-staple Egyptian cotton are needed by tire manufacturers. Every bit of this must be fumigated. Fear of cottonseeds infested with pink bollworm entering this country from Mexico necessitates similar treatment of 4,000 railroad cars a year. This is done in huge sheds that can handle as many as 20 cars at a time. The quarantine service examines 5,000 inbound planes per year and delves through half a million parcel post packages.

Certain crops—cane, wheat, cotton, potatoes, citrus—are completely excluded from some countries because of insect and disease plagues. Such importations as are made for propagation purposes are made only by the Federal Government. Extraordinary precautions attend them. Let us suppose that a Florida orchardist is particularly anxious to get cuttings from a Spanish orange tree to test with his own stock. He makes his wish known to the government, which volunteers to handle the importation.

Arrangements are made and the cuttings, carefully sealed, of course, go directly to the federal greenhouse at Glenn Dale, Maryland. Packages are opened in an isolation ward, triple-sealed by screen and glass from the outside world. For two years or more cuttings grow in this ward, subject to inspection by pathologists, entomologists and horticulturists. If they look safe after this period of isolation cuttings go to propogation houses. But as a precautionary measure the original import material is always destroyed. Similar stations are maintained for wheat at Sacaton, Arizona, and for sugar cane at Arlington Farm, Virginia.

A new station at Hoboken, New Jersey, is one of the world's most perfect inspection stations. Stock imported by nurserymen for propagation is examined here.

Skilled employees know about diseases prevalent at the point of origin of these plants and have reference books to refresh their memories. In addition, the department maintains a file containing 22,000 cards giving facts about pests which have not yet entered the United States. Hence inspectors know what they are looking for when geraniums come from Germany, or hyacinths from Holland.

At the Hoboken port of entry, plants undergo fumigation

in great tanks that can be flooded with hydrocyanic-acid gas. A hot-water dip kills the eel worms that infest certain bulbs, and refrigeration kills eggs and larvae of fruit flies. Fear of epidemics among orchids and azaleas doesn't prompt these precautions so much as fear ·that diseases damaging to food crops and forests will slip in with flowers. The Japanese beetle, recall, entered with a shipment of irises.

Routine examination of luggage at port and border stations frequently turns up material that might well be regarded as dynamite. A motorist returning home from Mexico had an innocent-looking water can strapped to the running board of his car. Thought his radiator might need a drink, he explained. To keep water from sloshing out he had stuck a potato over the spout.

An inspector cut the potato open and found it infested with *Epicaerus cognatus*—a fearfully destructive weevil. In its adult stage, this insect sprouts wings and can travel long distances. Had the motorist been allowed to carry this insect on to his California home the farm population might have paid millions for his unintentional mistake.

Another time a man was apprehended in Baltimore. He had just returned from South America and had a box of wood samples—he was a furniture manufacturer. The inspector found a few handfuls of cottonseeds in the bottom of the box. The man explained that he was taking these South American varieties back to his home in the Mississippi Delta. The seeds were crawling with larvae of the pink bollworm! If they had got through it is thoroughly possible that annual damage resulting would have amounted to millions. With a nice salute to detective fiction this went down on the records as the Pandora's Box Case.

For obvious reasons these examinations are frequently more rigid than those made by the customs service. The concealed trinket on which a returning traveler wishes to escape duty represents no very great loss to the government. But a bit of diseased or insect-ridden vegetable matter that slips through can cause damage that will extend through the rest of our history.

Inspectors are trained to look everywhere and expect almost anything. The bedding the Mexican field worker wants to carry across the border looks safe enough. But a few contaminated cottonseeds in the stuffing of a quilt can spell disaster in Texas cotton fields. A bit of bark on a piece of rustic furniture can carry a beetle that spreads Dutch elm disease; a few innocent-looking mangoes can harbor a destructive fruit fly; and an avocado seed can carry weevils capable of blotting out a lusty new orchard industry.

There are something like 40,000 pests in the world that have not as yet entered this country. Germany's nun moth is worse than the gypsy moth which we already have. We don't have the Asiatic rice-stem borer to ravage the South's rice crop; nor the peanut mosaic from Africa, which might destroy Virginia's big stake in this crop. The brown rust from Argentina is as yet safely excluded from the potato fields of Maine; and Italy's powdery mildew hasn't gotten into Kentucky's tobacco fields.

Pests occasionally enter the country despite all precautions. Then the domestic quarantine service attempts to bottle them up in a given area. It posts inspectors along roads leading from the quarantine belt to stop all cars and search for prohibited vegetable material. Meanwhile a heroic campaign of extermination goes on.

Such measures are occasionally successful. The Mediterranean fruit fly was completely exterminated in Florida a few years ago. The European corn borer escaped to make further state-border restrictions pointless. Efforts are now being made to stop the spread of the gypsy moth from New England, the white-fringed beetle from the Gulf Coast and the Japanese beetle from a well-defined area centering in New Jersey.

The quarantine service's job is to see that all these pests stay where they are. It is a good plan to take an understanding attitude when a highway inspector asks for the bunch of flowers you are taking from one state to another, or for the remains of the bon-voyage basket that someone thoughtfully sent you when you sailed for home. This slight cooperation may save millions of dollars for people whom you have never seen.

Once an insect pest is established in the country there are two weapons against him: poison and predatory enemies. The airplane, which can spread insecticides quickly and effectively is agriculture's newest adjunct. For the men who fly these planes, aviation is still in the dawn patrol days.

With heavy loads, they must fly three to six feet above the ground, facing perils every inch of the way: telephone lines, high-tension wires, stumps. To survive, the pilots must be infinitely skillful and coolheaded.

To get a better idea of the dangers involved let's ride with one of the pilots assigned to dust a series of small cotton fields. Finding the field is the first job and it isn't an easy one. From the air cotton looks very much alike and pilots have been known to dust fields miles away from the ones assigned them.

But we find the one we want and action starts. The field is hemmed in by trees. We dive in, the wheels of the plane rustling the leaves. For a split second it looks as if we must surely crash, but at the last moment the pilot pulls the plane up sharply. At the same instant he gives his engine full throttle. The sudden surge of power blasts the insecticide back on the cotton at the very edge of the trees. This maneuver is important because boll weevils hibernate in underbrush and always destroy the cotton at the edge of a field first.

After this initial dive we level off and streak across the field, flying a foot or two above the cotton and keeping at an even speed of about 100 miles per hour. The sensation isn't like that of stunt flying. There you are high enough for the ground to seem remote and harmless; here it is a hard reality almost within reaching distance.

The cloud of dust spraying from the plane covers a swath of cotton about 40 feet wide. Directly in front of us is another wall of trees. We head for it full tilt. At the last second the pilot pulls up sharply and we miss it by a few feet. We've finished one row and must reverse our path to dust the next one.

There are other perils ahead. A couple of trees jut from the middle of a field. Obviously, there isn't space enough between them to accommodate the wingspread of the plane, yet the pilot heads for them hell-for-leather. ("The cotton between them had to be dusted, didn't it?" he will inquire later.) As they rush toward us, he deftly tilts the wings and we squeeze through with only inches to spare on each side.

When we have finished our cargo of insecticide, we head back to the bumpy landing field for more. Trained Negro crews hoist it up and dump it into the bin. They load 600 pounds of insecticide into the plane. It takes fifteen minutes for the plane to unload it on the crops.

By this time the sun is just coming over the trees. Visibility couldn't be worse. The great ball of fire on the horizon blinds the pilot as he flies into it. Possibly it is blanking out a tree stump that rises seven or eight feet out of the field. Or perhaps it is obscuring the high-tension wires we must fly under.

Both have taken their toll of good pilots.

But there is no time to ask about those things. There is cotton to be dusted and dusted quickly. Once the hot sun has eaten the dew off the plants, there is nothing to hold the insecticide.

By ten o'clock we have finished the morning's work. We have dusted six hundred acres. At dusk when the dew returns we'll dust another four hundred acres—making 1,000 acres for the day. That isn't bad when you consider that a man on the ground working with a hand duster can handle only eight acres; and that the better power machines can handle only a hundred.

There are scores of risks to crop dusting beyond the ones

already recounted. If sulphur is being used an engine back-fire can ignite this highly explosive substance.

Birds knock holes in wings. An engine failure on a turn can cause a crash, and county telephone lines are always waiting to foul the undercarriage and drag a plane from the air.

All these things are accepted as normal hazards of the most hazardous business in the world.

Only the most competent crop-dusting pilots, working for the best-equipped companies, can get life insurance. Even then, their premiums are six times as high as those paid by a commercial airline pilot.

In a few hours vast areas of swamp can be salted down with Paris green to control malaria mosquitoes—a job that would take weeks or months done from boats. Grassless and treeless land that has eroded can be seeded from the air; and foresters in slow-moving autogiros can spot diseased trees.

Planting crops by plane is a practice of rising importance. Floodgates that admit water to rice fields are usually opened after the seed has been placed on dry ground. Using a plane, seed may be planted directly into flooded fields—thus insuring quick germination. Vetch, and other crops that return nitrogen to the soil, can be planted from the air while soil-exhausting crops like cotton are still standing.

Orchards, cranberry bogs, blueberry patches and vegetable crops can be dusted from the air to kill insects. But cotton receives most attention for the simple reason that it is the most pest-ridden of all crops.

The plane is fast and can work immediately after a downpour—when ground equipment would bog down. It is after such rains that boll weevils, army worms, and flea hoppers are most destructive.

Elementary physics explains the completeness of the job the plane accomplishes. The dust from the hopper is agitated and projected outward by the slip stream of the propeller at a speed of about 300 miles an hour.

Highly agitated, and lacking contact with the ground, each particle in this cloud takes on a positive electric charge and is thus repellent to every other particle. Cotton, in contact with the earth, carries a negative charge and actually attracts the particles.

One duster offered to buy drinks for a group of planters if they could find a *single* leaf in the field without its quota of poison.

Yet another method of controlling insect pests is to find that pest's natural enemy. Hundreds of American agricultural crops came from other countries. Insects which prey on these crops came along with their hosts, but parasites which attack the insects were left behind. With nature's superb system of checks and balances thus upset, destructive insects had no enemy to impede their extravagant multiplication. Hence a worldwide hunt for the parasites.

Curtis Clausen leads this hunt for the U.S. Department of Agriculture. He is baldish, blue-eyed, mild-mannered. For 25 years he has traveled almost constantly: through Sumatra, Manchuria, Kashmir, and remote South Sea Islands.

His enemies are formidable. Insect pests do about $2,000,-000,000 damage a year to U.S. crops.

Clausen's job—and the job of the eleven men under him—is to search out parasites which the insects left behind in their native countries, to capture and colonize them, and set them to work. This type of control has been far more effective than the use of poison sprays, and its first cost is its last.

The Division of Foreign Parasite Introduction maintains a permanent station at Yokohama. There is a second station at St. Cloud, outside Paris, closed because of war. From these centers periodic bug-hunting expeditions go out to remote corners of the earth.

There are something like half a million classified insects. Searching out from among this enormous population the desired parasite, ofttimes so minute that it is barely visible, is a job demanding patience and keen detective work. One of Clausen's expeditions will illustrate how it is done.

He was in Japan in 1920 when the order went out to find a killer bug for the Japanese beetle. Armed with a hand lens and a few cotton-stoppered test tubes, Clausen started north into the orchard country. Here, he knew, the beetles were present but offered no problem. Some parasite held them in check.

Near Sapporo, examining adult beetles, he found, firmly attached to the body of one of them, a nest of minute white eggs. Clausen was thoroughly familiar with this old parasite trick, a means of providing food for the young. When eggs hatched, larvae wriggled forth, bored their way into the host's body and ate it hollow. But, to identify the parasite, he would have to watch the eggs hatch, and allow the larvae to grow.

He quickly set up a field laboratory and announced that he would pay 25 cents for each 100 beetles carrying such egg masses. Attracted by visions of sudden wealth, 200 children collected 100,000 beetles in a single day.

The parasite, it turned out, might easily be mistaken for the common housefly. In a week's time this potent killer would destroy 90 per cent of the beetles in an orchard. Clausen dispatched shipments of his parasite to the United States. But here, for some reason—perhaps climatic—the fly's life cycle no longer synchronized with the beetle's. The fly emerged a month early and its days were over before the beetle crawled out from hibernation.

Clausen set out again, this time with success. He found two minute wasps which, seeking out the beetle grubs underground, stung their prey into a state of paralysis, then attached eggs to their bodies. Hatched larvae ate the grubs. These wasps are now being colonized along the Atlantic Seaboard with promising results.

One of Clausen's outstanding jobs was finding the parasite

for the Cuban black fly. This pest was eating foliage, stunting fruit and killing trees in Cuban orchards. The U.S. Department of Agriculture feared it might jump to Florida and endanger the state's $2,000,000,000 citrus industry. Clausen took ship for Singapore and started working his way through the citrus orchards of the Malay States.

After months of labor he found a wasp, even more minute than the gnat-sized black fly. This wasp punctured the body of the black fly and inserted her eggs. When the hatched larvae were through feeding, the black fly was a hollow shell.

Discovering this harsh little drama of nature was only a start. How get the short-lived wasps to Cuba? Several generations would eat, breed and die in the time required for the voyage. Clausen would have to provide black flies for the parasites to eat, and, in turn, something for the black flies themselves to eat.

Clausen packed hundreds of potted mango seedlings tightly in a dozen screened cases. He stocked each case heavily with black flies—enough, he hoped, to outlast the wasps. The shipment got through—just. All the flies were dead but 40 parasites arrived—enough, it proved, to populate the island, erase Cuba's plague, and remove a threat to the United States.

Altogether, scattered through the world, there have been 25 examples of insects being brought under complete control by parasites. The first and greatest was the cottony cushion scale which late last century devastated California citrus fruit. Orchards were being abandoned and bankruptcy threatened whole communities when Albert Koebele, a self-trained entomologist, started on a dramatically successful expedition.

The scale, Koebele knew, was taking a terrible toll in the orchards of New Zealand. But it was no problem in Australia, the source of New Zealand's nursery stock. Apparently the parasite had been left behind when trees and scale were shipped to New Zealand and the search should begin in Australia. Koebele sailed in the fall of 1888. In an amazingly short time he found a small beetle which laid its eggs on top of the egg masses of the cottony cushion scale. When the beetle eggs hatched, larvae crawled out to consume the scale eggs.

Koebele managed to get 129 of his parasites back to California alive. In a year's time millions of descendants had completely controlled the pest. Subsequently shipments of the parasite have erased the plague from 40 countries.

Two of our parasitic newcomers work well against the European corn borer in New England, and another against the satin moth on the Pacific Coast. Why don't they work as well in other regions? No one knows. A fly which arrived on the first commercial trip of the transatlantic clipper appears to be highly efficient against the asparagus beetle. And good results are coming from a parasite for the spruce sawfly—the insect which, in one recent year, destroyed enough trees in Canada and New England to keep pulp mills running for a quarter of a century.

New problems are always arising. The white-fringed beetle, for example, appeared in Florida three years ago, apparently from the Argentine, and has spread along the Gulf Coast all the way to Louisiana. In four hours one man in a badly infested area collected 80,000! As a grub living underground it eats roots of plants, and as an adult it destroys whatever vegetation is left on the surface. Another ominous threat is the pink bollworm which slipped across the Rio Grande into the cotton fields of Texas.

Search for parasites for both these pests is under way. The work of Clausen's band of hunters has been speeded up tremendously by the advent of transoceanic plane service. Parasites which formerly required tedious nursemaiding and frequent stopovers can now be shipped directly to receiving stations in New Jersey, Connecticut, Pennsylvania and Oregon. About 30 promising new species enter the United States each year. Climatic, nutritional and other conditions kill some off. But to date 70-odd new species have thrived in their new home, and are doing their part in reestablishing nature's balance which man upset. Many times over they have paid the cost of maintaining the globe-trotting bug hunters.